THE NEW
PARKINSON'S
TREATMENT

EXERCISE IS MEDICINE

Melissa McConaghy, FACP

First published 2014 for Melissa McConaghy by

Publish-*Me!*

PO Box 205 Haberfield NSW 2045
www.publish-me.com.au
info@publish-me.com.au
T. +61 2 9362 8441

For the National Library of Australia Cataloguing-in-Publication entry, please see www.nla.gov.au.

ISBN: 9780994386311

Melissa McConaghy

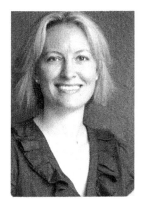

Melissa McConaghy FACP holds a Master of Health Science in Neurological Physiotherapy and is one of seven Specialist Neurological Physiotherapists in Australia. She became the youngest Fellow of the Australian College of Physiotherapists in 2010. She is the past Chair and National Representative of the NSW Neurology Group for the Australian Physiotherapy Association.

Melissa is a passionate advocate for exercise and rehabilitation and is the Managing Director and founder of Advance Rehab Centre and PD Warrior, both based in Sydney.

About PD Warrior

Melissa developed PD Warrior, an Australian first, with her colleague, Lynn Tullock, over an exciting two-year period of researching, modelling, and testing the latest scientific evidence regarding neuroplasticity and exercise. Lynn is a neurological physiotherapist and Clinical Director of the Advance Rehab Centre. Since 2001, she has had a special interest in the field of neurological rehabilitation, particularly Parkinson's.

Contents

Introduction: How you live with Parkinson's is up to you vii

1. Parkinson's in a Nutshell 1
2. Traditional Approaches to Treatment 12
3. The PD Warrior Revolution 21
4. PD Warrior Principles 35
5. Things to Consider before Doing PD Warrior 49
6. How to Get Started 57
7. Common Misperceptions 69
8. How to Stay Motivated 76
9. The 10-Week Challenge 90
10. PD Warrior Core Exercises 112
11. Life after PD Warrior 150

Record and Assessment Sheets 155
    10-Week Challenge 155
    Assessment Measures 166
    PDQ-8 Questionnaire 167
    Berg Balance Scale 168
    Self-Assessment PD Disease Scale 171
    Activity Log 173
    Goals 174
    Performance Graph 175

References 176

Disclaimer

The aim of this publication is to provide information of a general nature across a variety of general settings, situations, and circumstances. The information herein is intended only as a guide and does not provide specific advice or replace advice provided to you by your medical professional or other specialist in the area.

This book is written on the understanding that the author is not engaged in rendering medical services and that the book is not providing advice for specific situations. Specific medical advice should be sought by any suffering from Parkinson's before implementing anything in this book.

The author and the publishing services providor accept no responsibility or liability for the actions of any person who may use the information in this publication.

Introduction

How you live with Parkinson's is up to you

The intention of *The New Parkinson's Treatment: Exercise is Medicine* is to introduce you and other interested parties to a revolutionary new approach to the treatment of Parkinson's called PD Warrior.

Neurologists and other health professionals are referring to PD Warrior as a 'game-changer' and, since its launch in Sydney, Australia, in April 2012, it has grown exponentially, with extremely successful outcomes and widespread popularity.

The philosophy behind PD Warrior is that exercise, education, community, and a life-long commitment to fighting the symptoms of Parkinson's cannot be underestimated. If you have Parkinson's and you are not doing PD Warrior, you are likely missing out. PD Warrior gives you an opportunity to fight the symptoms of your disease and to slow the progression down, to take control of the disease and your life.

The book is designed for:

- People with Parkinson's who are curious about the potential of PD Warrior
- People already doing PD Warrior who want to learn more about the theory underpinning the program

- Family and friends of people with Parkinson's
- Health professionals interested in becoming certified
  PD Warrior Instructors

The aim of PD Warrior is to help you develop a greater state of physical, mental, and social wellbeing. If you have recently been diagnosed with Parkinson's, you are not alone - thirty people are diagnosed with Parkinson's every day in Australia and the number is rising by about four per cent each year. There is currently no cure, but it is rarely terminal. Parkinson's is simply a condition that you live with. How well you live with it is determined by whether you are at your best throughout the different stages of the condition.

Traditional approaches to managing Parkinson's have improved vastly over the last few decades. It was in the 1960s that Levodopa medication was first introduced, and it changed entirely the landscape of how Parkinson's is managed and treated. Since then, apart from neurosurgical techniques, such as pallidotomy and deep brain stimulation, there have been relatively few breakthroughs in therapy and management.

Until now ...

In the last few years, there has been a growing body of evidence showing that exercise may play a fundamental role in protecting the brain and stimulating the most efficient movement pathways possible. It is this capacity for the brain to re-organise itself and learn, called neuroplasticity, that lies at the heart of PD Warrior. PD Warrior is a sophisticated combination of intensive physical and mental exercises that harnesses the brain's 'plasticity' to help you to move better. It may also have an effect at the cellular level on disease progression. Exercise is medicine, and when prescribed correctly, it is an incredibly powerful tool.

The New Parkinson's Treatment: Exercise is Medicine is a must read if you have been newly diagnosed with Parkinson's or are in the early stages. PD Warrior has given people hope that there is indeed life - quality of life - after a diagnosis of Parkinson's. Parkinson's once robbed people of their independence, dignity, and enjoyment of life. Today, the situation is quite different and your approach to living with Parkinson's is pivotal to your wellbeing - maintaining mobility and cognitive function are absolute priorities.

As a neurological physiotherapist, I have been treating people with Parkinson's since 2000 and have seen the very dark days some experience. It doesn't have to be that way. PD Warrior is not a cure and doesn't propose to be one. What it is, is very hard work, but often with amazing results. In all the years I have spent treating people with Parkinson's, I have never seen results from any other treatment equal those achieved with PD Warrior.

This book strives to answer the most common questions people ask about their diagnosis and how PD Warrior can make a difference. Examples of these questions, which will be discussed in greater depth further on, include:

1. What does a diagnosis of Parkinson's mean?

Being diagnosed with Parkinson's can be a terrifying experience, especially when combined with misinformation and a graphic imagination. Most of you probably merit a doctorate in Google searching by this stage! This book helps put this diagnosis in perspective and demonstrates that, from here on out, how someone responds to being diagnosed with this condition will determine more about its progression than anything else.

2. What options do I have for treatment?

Traditional therapy for Parkinson's has revolved largely around medication and compensatory movement strategies. For a select few, brain surgery has also been recommended. PD Warrior challenges the status quo and promotes exercise as medicine as an early intervention strategy. Used in combination with optimal medication dosing, PD Warrior has shown dramatically superior results versus traditional therapy and medication alone.

3. My symptoms are still really mild; do I really need to do PD Warrior?

Most often, even in the very mild stages of Parkinson's, people have already started to modify their life around their disease: subconsciously avoiding social activities, modifying the clothes they wear to avoid buttons and zippers, changing the food they order in restaurants – subtle adaptations they may not even be aware of. Without treatment, they will continue to give up the things they enjoy. PD Warrior can help you to recognise these signs and, most important, learn how to fight the symptoms and get back into life. Think hard. What have you already given up?

4. Is exercise helpful for people with Parkinson's?

New research in basic neuroscience reveals that exercise may be the only ammunition we currently have to slow down the development of symptoms. However, general exercise by itself is unlikely to be sufficient to slow the symptoms of Parkinson's down. Instead, precise exercises targeting the symptoms need to be the focus. This book provides a step-by-step exercise program specifically designed and shown to improve the quality of life and movement for people with early-stage Parkinson's.

The New Parkinson's Treatment: Exercise is Medicine is the collaboration of the current literature available with nearly two years of clinical practice and modelling and feedback gained from the PD Warriors themselves who have truly shaped PD Warrior. Although based heavily on the science and evidence, this book has simplified the concepts to make for easy, straightforward reading. If you are interested in the specifics in the literature, there is a comprehensive reference list provided in the back of the book.

5. How do I get started with PD Warrior?

The New Parkinson's Treatment: Exercise is Medicine is a clear guide outlining precautions to exercise, what equipment and space is required, how to stay motivated, and helpful hints and tips to get started. PD Warrior is understandably best begun with an onsite assessment performed by a certified PD Warrior Instructor (http://www.pdwarrior.com/locations) and being introduced to the PD Warrior principles and the core exercises through several one-on-one sessions with an instructor; however, this book enables you to effect your own do-it-yourself (DIY) program.

The New Parkinson's Treatment: Exercise is Medicine discusses the traditional experience and treatment of Parkinson's and introduces you, the reader, to the innovative perspective and approach of PD Warrior. It is recommended that you read it cover to cover before doing the *10-Week Challenge*, because understanding the principles of PD Warrior is necessary to ensure a safe and successful outcome.

6. How will I know if it's working?

The crux of PD Warrior is its *10-Week Challenge*. (You will learn more about this in Chapter 9.) If performed correctly, it can produce stunning results. The PD Warrior framework in this book provides instructions and self-assessment techniques that you can use to evaluate and record your progress as you work through the program.

You will know it is working when you can feel yourself moving better, doing things that you had lost the confidence doing, rewarding yourself for achieving your goals, and when other people start commenting on your progress.

7. What other health professionals should I be working with?

The earlier you enlist the help of health professionals familiar with your symptoms, issues, and goals, the sooner you can get back into life. There is a range of people you can include in your medical team, and a multidisciplinary approach is the best approach in my experience. You do not need to meet with all of them, and many of those with whom you do will be necessary only for annual check-ups. It is important that if you are having difficulties, you recognise them early and get the right help immediately. Your PD Warrior Instructor can refer you to a local health professional or community service as appropriate.

Your Team

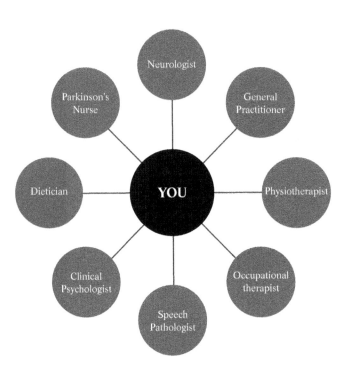

Special thanks

Thank you to all the PD Warriors who have participated in the development of the program, for all the questionnaires we asked you to fill in, all the hours of exercise we made you do, and all the time you spent supporting the development of the program. Special mention to Cindy Summers and her husband Michael for all your advice and extra time in helping to get PD Warrior off the ground. I would also like to thank Dr Stephen Tisch for his support in helping us on our journey.

Although the comments, thoughts, and opinions in this book are mine, I would like to thank Lynn Tullock for co-developing the PD Warrior program with me. Without her expertise, enthusiasm, and brilliant ideas, PD Warrior would not be the success it is today.

To Gilly Davy, Aimee Barnes, Alison Wighton, Lyndsay Hendry, and Emma Lee, the dedicated team of neurological physiotherapists at Advance Rehab Centre, thank you for being the sounding board and clinical instructors we needed to help us to develop the program further.

To my wonderful husband and family, thank you for your unending support and the hours you have let me prattle on long into the night.

Finally, my thanks to you, the reader, for taking the time to read this book. I sincerely hope that PD Warrior is a positive experience for you. Most importantly, if you have been diagnosed with Parkinson's, I hope it gives you a healthy perspective on having Parkinson's and the confidence to get back into life.

This is your chance to take control and be part of the PD Warrior Revolution!

The *'Parka'*
The PD Warrior War Cry

'Parkinson's, Parkinson's, STOP!

Use it, improve it.

Be big, be strong.

Parkinson's, Parkinson's, STOP!'

1

Parkinson's in a Nutshell

'You might have Parkinson's, but does it have you?'
Dr Simon Lewis

What does a diagnosis of Parkinson's mean?

If you are reading this book, then you or someone you know has recently been diagnosed with Parkinson's. Myriad thoughts will run through your mind – that is, if you have managed to push through the fog of uncertainty.

Many of the people who come to me confess having felt, at the time of diagnosis, uncertain about their future. Their greatest fear is often losing control: losing control of their current lifestyle, of their movements, and even of their thoughts and memory. I can tell you right now that, on the whole, your imagination of what it means to have this disease is often far worse than the disease itself.

The Cause and Effect of Parkinson's

To understand how to address Parkinson's, it's helpful to first understand something about its pathology, its cause and effects. True Parkinson's is called *idiopathic* Parkinson's. Idiopathic indicates Parkinson's that has arisen spontaneously and without known cause. The reason this is important is that, although your symptom presentation will differ from that of the next person, the underlying pathology is the same. A positive feature of idiopathic Parkinson's is that you typically respond well to medication, and to PD Warrior!

There is currently no blood screening, MRI, X-ray, or fancy test that can definitively tell you whether you have idiopathic Parkinson's, however, your doctor or neurologist will be confident of a diagnosis based on three things: your symptoms, your response to medication, and the exclusion of other neurological conditions. That doesn't mean you won't undergo several tests - most doctors and neurologists run these in order to exclude other neurological conditions.

You may present with all or perhaps just one of these clinical symptoms: **rigidity** or stiffness in the muscles and joints; **tremor** that comes on when you are resting; slow movements (called **bradykinesia)**. About a third of people first notice issues that are not related to poor movement, such as constipation, loss of smell, or loss of short-term memory. Your spouse may complain of your nocturnal violence - involuntary thrashing when you sleep at night. Everyone with Parkinson's is different, and you will have a different journey from the next person. What may be similar is how one or more of the symptoms of Parkinson's affects your movements.

Clinicians commonly define bradykinesia and rigidity as 'poverty of movement.' Technically, that means being unable to generate the correct amount of motor output required to initiate and drive normal movement. It can feel like being slow to both start moving and being slow *when* you move. Difficulty with dexterity, such as doing up buttons, losing the body's natural arm swing when walking, or developing a stiff, rigid posture, can all be a direct result of this

2

overall poverty of movement, specifically when you aren't producing sufficient **dopamine** in a particular part of your brain.

For reasons that are still unknown, the cells in a part of the brain called the *substantia nigra,* which are responsible for producing dopamine in the basal ganglia (involved in coordinating movement), start to die off in people with Parkinson's.

The basal ganglia sit roughly in the middle of your brain. I like to think of it as our switchboard. The basal ganglia regulate movement after receiving input from those parts of the brain that initiate movement. If you have less dopamine in your system, the net result is that your movements will become slower and smaller, with less control. If you increase the amount of dopamine in the system through medication, your movement will improve significantly.

If medication can do that, isn't that enough? Why should I worry about doing anything else?

Despite medication, your body starts to recalibrate over time – your body starts to move less – producing smaller, slower movements, which becomes normal to you. This learned non-use and re-sizing of your movements is best described with this analogy: think about what happens when you take your foot off your car's accelerator pedal. It slows down. The fuel is no longer driving the engine forward. It's the same when your body learns to move with smaller movements. In the early stages of Parkinson's, more often than not, you can still achieve movements that look 'normal', but your brain has already begun learning to take your foot off the accelerator pedal (with or without medication). To a point, the medication will improve your movements, but it will not teach you to put your foot back down on the accelerator pedal. This is important for many reasons.

The progression of Parkinson's

At diagnosis, most of the cells producing dopamine have already been destroyed, in some cases up to 70 per cent. It is only once this threshold has been reached that the common symptoms of Parkinson's become evident. As it progresses, more and more of these cells die, leading to further poverty of movement and difficulty with more and more tasks, all of which are often associated with behavioural and cognitive changes. Currently, medication can help remedy dopamine deficiency; however, to date, it has been unable to protect the dopamine-producing cells from continued destruction. We need a sufficient number of these cells in order to distribute the dopamine our bodies need. When Parkinson's is left unchecked, there is only a small window of time in which medication can have a positive effect before there are no longer enough receptor cells to receive the simulated dopamine, let alone naturally produce it.

There are significant side effects associated with taking medication that should not be taken lightly. These need to be considered in your Parkinson's management plan - not as a justification not to take medication, but as a reason why it cannot be taken to the exclusion of all other treatment options. We talk more about this in Chapter 2.

Due to the progressive nature of cell destruction in Parkinson's, strategies known to protect the dopamine-producing cells that remain, slow the destruction of further cells, and enhance the brain's natural ability to re-wire itself are at the centre of finding a cure for Parkinson's.

Until recently, this progression of cell death was considered irreversible and could not be slowed. Although Parkinson's is currently still incurable, new evidence suggests there is the potential to modify the disease progression and slow the emergence of symptoms and, in the early stages, clinically reverse them with exercise.

New evidence suggests there is the potential to modify the disease progression and slow the emergence of symptoms and, in the early stages, clinically reverse them with exercise.

The evidence that exercise is neuro-protective and can stop your dopamine producing cells from dying off is by no means conclusive. What is conclusive is that exercise can teach our brains how to learn. Exercise can teach your brain how to put its foot back down on the accelerator pedal and work harder to drive normal movement. This

4

is the focus of PD Warrior and our research over the last few years. This principle is called *neuroplasticity*.

Neuroplasticity is not a new concept in neurological rehabilitation. We have been applying this concept in rehabilitation for over twenty years. It is, however, a new concept in the way we manage Parkinson's. For that reason, PD Warrior is one of the first programs to use this model of therapy and why it is so exciting.

Impact of Parkinson's on function, behaviour, and emotion

Parkinson's not only makes physical activities and daily function more difficult; it also has an impact on a whole range of behaviours, moods, and emotions. Common behavioural and emotional issues seen in Parkinson's include apathy, depression, anxiety, and introversion (social withdrawal). One or all of these problems can lead to reduced social participation and a more limited lifestyle.

Apathy

Apathy (not to be confused with depression) is common in many people with Parkinson's. Apathy is described as a distinct loss of interest, or detachment. I see this often when a loved one brings in a potential client, wanting them to start an exercise program. The problem with true apathy is that you are just not interested in participating in anything, especially an exercise program, no matter how much your spouse or family may want you to. As a physiotherapist, my job is to encourage and motivate people to exercise, even when they don't want to. Over the years I have developed tools and tricks that are quite persuasive; however, in my experience, it is very hard to help someone make significant changes in their life if they are not inspired to do so themselves because of severe apathy.

If you feel a certain level of indifference to your current situation and are not interested in improving your health, you may not be ready for PD Warrior. Your GP, neurologist, or a psychiatrist may be able to help you further, especially in determining whether your apathy is directly related to Parkinson's or a side effect of depression.

Depression

Depression is probably the most common psychiatric disorder observed in Parkinson's. It is estimated that up to 50 per cent of people with Parkinson's will experience a major depressive episode lasting at least two weeks. Depression can be caused by Parkinson's directly or be due to the grief relating to the change in life circumstances, frustration at the decreasing levels of function and ability, helplessness at the decreasing overall quality of life, and mood change related to increasingly sedentary behaviour.

Depression can be difficult to recognise in people with Parkinson's as many of the physical signs of depression - reduced facial expression, loss of interest in hobbies or work, poor sleeping habits, for example - are common with Parkinson's, even when the individual does not suffer from depression. There is also a school of thought that says if you look depressed, you will start to feel depressed. This certainly does not help the matter.

Depression can have as marked an effect on disability as motor problems in Parkinson's, if not more. If you feel persistent depression, please seek advice from your GP or neurologist before starting PD Warrior. Although exercise has been linked to improved mood and shown to have a treatment effect on depression, you will get a lot more out of this program, and ultimately out of your life, if you are actively managing any symptoms of depression.

Anxiety

It is common, although not a rule, that depression and anxiety often go hand in hand with Parkinson's. Anxiety in this context applies to feelings of inappropriate disquiet or irrational alarm and can be very debilitating. I often treat patients who report extreme anxiety, which limits them leaving the house or walking in crowded areas such as shopping centres or busy streets. Many of my patients report never having had feelings of depression or anxiety prior to diagnosis. There are some reports that anxiety may also be medication-related. Discussion with your neurologist and GP before starting this program may help you to manage your symptoms.

Treatment can involve changing your medications or prescribing counselling. Either way, in my experience, the anxiety seen in Parkinson's can be greatly improved through PD Warrior. I have seen firsthand how PD Warrior has helped participants regain their confidence and the control they once felt was slipping away from them. Lack of control is a fear I hear a lot of people admit before they start the program. Some of my clients report that it is their subsequent increased confidence and ability to manage their symptoms that helps to reduce their anxiety as much as the physical aspects of the program. I am not suggesting PD Warrior is a cure for anxiety, but it can help.

There seems to be an unfortunate – and undeserved – stigma attached to seeking counselling services in Australia. The best athletes don't hesitate to hire sports psychologists to help them achieve and be their best. Think of yourself as an athlete – a PD Warrior athlete. To be your best, you need a coach to help you achieve that best. Counselling in conjunction with PD Warrior is an excellent way to combat feelings of anxiety and depression.

Introversion

Introversion and associated social isolation can be a significant problem in Parkinson's, regardless of whether the primary cause is physical disability, mood or behavioural change, or a combination of these. How many times in the last month have you declined a social invitation? Be honest. Take a little time to reflect on why you said no. Did you feel a perceived physical limitation that would have prevented you from enjoying the event? Did you feel that you couldn't be bothered? Was it too frustrating to think you might not be able to participate? Did you feel embarrassed or ashamed about what people might think of you? Perhaps you haven't told anyone that you have Parkinson's and didn't want to be caught out.

Think back over the last three months - how much of life have you given up?

Are you ready to get your life back?

How you deal with the diagnosis from here on

I was diagnosed with Parkinson's disease six or seven years ago. Initially I was relieved to find out what was wrong with me but my wife was very upset at the time.

I was told to take the tablets and come back in a month. If they worked, then I had Parkinson's disease. I had no understanding of the condition. I thought Parkinson's was just shaking. I didn't have any understanding of the full ramifications of the disease, how it progressed, or how to control the symptoms. It was a hard time for me because I was given no information and nothing to read.

I have always exercised, all my life - born and bred. I love the feeling of excitement, the rush of blood in your veins, and I believe it is a dopamine maker. The more you do it, the more you want it.
– Peter Marshall, PD Warrior

Recognising what you have lost, missed out on, or given up on in life can be incredibly challenging. I have been told that the PD Warrior program is one of the most confronting things some have ever done, because the person must face how far they have let things slide. Acknowledging this loss of ground is one of the crucial steps one must take in order to get back into life. Until you can recognise some of the key parts of your life that need to change - and I mean really change - your goals will remain insipid and lack conviction. You need to identify powerful goals that will keep driving you forward on your journey, despite the setbacks and the hard work. Until you realise that how you deal with your diagnosis from here is more about *you* than about your diagnosis, you will always have Parkinson's and, worse, it will always have you.

General Health

General exercise is crucial to good health. Having Parkinson's does not make you immune to other health concerns, such as heart or respiratory problems or blood sugar-related problems like diabetes. It has been proven that, if you simply give up because you have Parkinson's and adopt or continue with a sedentary lifestyle, you are much more likely to develop co-morbidities and other health problems that can make life much more challenging, and your symptoms of Parkinson's will likely accelerate.

The World Health Organisation (WHO) defined health in its broader sense in 1946 as 'a state of complete physical, mental, and social wellbeing and not merely the absence of disease or infirmity.' Now, whether there is any such thing as 'complete' physical, mental, and social wellbeing can be debated, but what I like about this statement is that your general health is more than the absence of poor health. It is your overall wellbeing, which is viewed as a very positive thing. Most people whom I assess initially are understandably focused on the progression of the disease and associated disability. The most common questions I get asked are: *What is my prognosis?* and *What do I do now?*

The PD Warrior program described in this book, *The New Parkinson's Treatment: Exercise is Medicine* is about helping you to develop a state of physical, mental, and social wellbeing, regardless of your Parkinson's. Most of the PD Warriors who complete the *10-Week Challenge* gain a real sense of wellbeing by the end of the program, and what is often most profound is a very real sense of empowerment. The people who put the most into the program definitely get the most out of it, not just in terms of fitness, mobility, and confidence scores, but in overall wellbeing.

> PD Warrior is a sophisticated combination of intensive physical and mental exercises that harnesses the brain's 'plasticity' to help you to move better.

According to the data from the 2012 report from the Australian Institute of Health and Welfare, Australians have one of the highest life expectancies in the world. Good on us Aussies! What is concerning perhaps is that 'People with disabilities aged under 65 are much more likely than people without disabilities to report having long-term physical and mental health conditions, and to rate their overall health as fair or poor'. With up to 20 per cent of the population newly diagnosed with Parkinson's under the age of 65, this data, although not surprising, is alarming.

Parkinson's in this day and age is never fatal; it is simply something you learn to live with. That is a very important distinction and one that is worthy of some consideration. Parkinson's is NOT a death sentence; however, how you manage your overall general health ultimately determines how *well* you live with Parkinson's. If you curl up in a ball and give in, Parkinson's could be the least of your problems.

> Parkinson's is not a death sentence.
> You determine how you live with it.

What is more misleading is some of the information related to Parkinson's in the Deloitte Access Economics data from 2011, stating that 'The median time from onset to death is 12.2 years, though many people with Parkinson's live with the disease for well over 20 years'. (p. ii). I think this statement overlooks the obvious point that most are in their sixties when diagnosed with Parkinson's. The average life expectancy in Australia is 79.5 years for males and 84 years for females. What accounts for the difference between time of death and average life expectancy likely has far more to do with general health and the morbidity associated with a sedentary lifestyle than merely the fact of having Parkinson's.

It is estimated that 52,000 people in Australia are in the early stages of Parkinson's, classified as mild to moderate. If this includes you, I hope that you have started to grasp the role that *you* play in how your Parkinson's progresses, and how *you* are going to manage it. No one cares about how your disease progresses as much as you do. There has never been a better time for you to access the information you need and rally the troops to start fighting Parkinson's.

I love this quote from singer/songwriter Garth Brooks: 'Every man dies, but not every man lives.' What do you think about when you read that statement? Are you living the best life you can? If not, what are you going to do about it?

To return to my original point about general health, maintaining peak general health is crucial in helping you to manage your Parkinson's. Trying to avoid a heart problem or diabetes by keeping fit and maintaining a good diet may put you in better shape than many of your couch potato peers who do not have Parkinson's.

2

Traditional Approaches to Treatment

'The intention to live as long as possible isn't one of the mind's best intentions, because quantity isn't the same as quality.'

Deepak Chopra

Traditional approaches to treatment

Having worked as a physiotherapist since 2000, I have treated many people with Parkinson's over the years. Before developing PD Warrior, I worked with people with Parkinson's regularly and I remember feeling somewhat redundant, as it was one of the few conditions I felt there was little I could do.

At both undergraduate and master's levels at university, I was taught ways to use compensatory movement strategies to help people: using external cueing ideas, such as lines on the floor in areas notorious for causing freezing; providing falls prevention advice, teaching people how to minimise environmental risk factors that might lead to freezing and falling; and even advice on how to teach people to stop and talk, and not walk and talk, at the same time.

The sad fact though was that, if the individual was freezing, the evidence indicated I couldn't successfully change this. If they were falling over, again the evidence indicated I couldn't stop them from falling. If they were struggling with everyday movements, medication alone would make the difference. There was nothing ground breaking to help people that I could sink my teeth into, and I considered rehab for people with Parkinson's a bit gloomy because of this.

At the other end of the spectrum, had I assessed someone who, these days, I would consider perfect for PD Warrior, back then I would have thought, 'Your symptoms are too mild; there's not much I can do for you either'. Tragic. Although I might have been up to date with current clinical practice, I was not up to date with the new body of evidence emerging to help people at this level. I was not alone. No one in Australia was treating people newly diagnosed with Parkinson's. We just didn't know how.

It is amazing how slowly clinical practice moves forward, even as the research uncovers more about how people respond to the condition – they say it can take up to 17 years. What I can say about the compensatory movement strategies we were taught is that, yes, they can be effective tools if you are further along in your Parkinson's journey. If you are already falling or freezing, then most physiotherapists will be aware of such strategies and how to implement them effectively. You will benefit from these traditional forms of therapy, but I believe there is so much more that we can offer now.

What these strategies do not address are the difficulties that you are likely to experience if you have been newly diagnosed with Parkinson's. If your symptoms are mild, it is unlikely you are falling, it is unlikely that you are freezing, and it is unlikely that you need to implement any of the compensatory strategies taught with traditional physiotherapy techniques. You might find it more challenging to drive, but you are probably still doing it, possibly still working, and certainly still talking and walking at the same time.

There are two reasons why teaching you traditional strategies at the mild stage is not appropriate: the first is that you are too competent for what these strategies offer; and the second is that you can improve on the difficulties you are experiencing using other, far more effective methods.

PD Warrior is one of the first approaches in Australia to address and treat the initial impairments of Parkinson's directly. Our approach is not to teach you ways to compensate for poor movement. We teach you how to *use it and improve it*, tackling your specific impairments head on by engaging the pathways and cells in your basal ganglia. We use principles of neuroplastic change so that you can help yourself to re-wire your brain to create more efficient pathways for better movement. The goal of PD Warrior is to help you move more freely and with greater confidence. We hope also to help you slow down symptom development.

PD Warrior is one of the first approaches in Australia to address and treat the initial impairments of Parkinson's directly. We teach you how to *use it and improve it*, tackling your specific impairments head on by engaging the pathways and cells in your basal ganglia.

Without looking into the latest literature, this may seem a radical concept to experienced physiotherapists who are very familiar with traditional approaches. Believe me, I had my own reservations when I started looking into the literature several years ago. However, the results speak for themselves. PD Warrior is a treatment style of the future and is part of a growing body of evidence that will re-write the teaching books in universities for young physiotherapists coming through in the next few years.

Medication

Rarely a day goes by when I am not asked the question 'Should I be taking medication?' If you are considering starting medication, this may be a question you are asking yourself on a regular basis. If you are currently taking medication, perhaps you have lingering doubts as to whether you should be taking it. In either scenario, my answer to this is the same. As a physiotherapist, my job is not to advise you on whether or not you should be taking medication – that is the purview of your GP or neurologist.

That said, while there are many reasons for and against taking medication, in most instances there are more reasons that support taking medication. For example, if you have started to notice difficulties in everyday activities, such as tying up your shoelaces, pulling on tight clothing, loss of confidence walking in crowded areas, and so on, then you may benefit from starting medication now.

There are many different types of medication, ranging from dopamine replacement therapies to those that block different types of chemicals in the brain from breaking down the available dopamine in your system. What most of these medications will help you with is improving your overall motor output and your capacity to resume doing activities you are starting to struggle with. The reason this is a good thing, I think, is pretty obvious. If you can keep doing the things that you love doing for longer, not only are you moving better, but you are also liable to participate in more social activities, which is great for your mood; you are probably exercising more, which maintains your fitness; and likely to be living each day more, which gives you a much better quality of life.

The flipside of taking medication for Parkinson's, however, is that it is not without side effects and some of these can be serious. Again, this is a very good reason why you should discuss the role of medication with your GP and/or neurologist carefully.

Deep brain stimulation (DBS)

DBS is a surgical procedure used to treat specific symptoms of Parkinson's. Most of the success in DBS has been seen in the reduction of tremor, dyskinesias, and the significant on/off periods that people experience. DBS can be very effective in returning independence and mobility to people with Parkinson's. It, too, is not without side effects and risk factors, not least of all because DBS involves major neurosurgery and all the possible complications associated with it. DBS is also only effective in about 10 to 15 per cent of the population of people with Parkinson's. It is mainly reserved for people who have responded well to medication, but are now plagued by severe dyskinesias, tremor, or large motor fluctuations, depending on the medication on/off periods.

Most doctors believe that DBS surgery may have only a five- to 10-year treatment effect and can only be performed once. DBS, it is believed, does not act directly on the dopamine-producing cells of the brain; instead, it compensates for the major effects of dopamine loss. The cells that produce dopamine still continue to perish after DBS.

Exercise

Exercise and exercise therapies have been used to treat people with Parkinson's for many decades. Most exercise programs designed for people with Parkinson's in my experience (prior to developing PD Warrior) assume that you need to be wrapped in cotton wool and are not capable of working hard. Perhaps because most programs are targeted at people who are in the later stages of Parkinson's and at greater risk of falls, many of the programs are designed to be performed at low intensity and, more often than not, in a seated position.

It is also unfortunate but people with Parkinson's are not referred to physiotherapy as frequently as they should be. If they are referred, it is usually after a fall, long after they have started to scale down their life, given up activities, and lost some independence. If you have had Parkinson's for some time now and have ever been prescribed an exercise program, the traditional approach would be to improve your strength, balance, flexibility, and function. There would also be a strong focus on preventing falls.

Russell Tuckerman, East Gosford Physiotherapist & PD Warrior Licensee, observed:

One significant issue I have found since working with PD patients is the de-conditioning that comes with a chronic disease, which excludes you from 'normal' exercise models. Traditionally, physios would give you a few balance and mobility exercises, but offer no fitness advice. The fitness industry of gyms and boot camps tend to exclude someone who is nervous, slow, and unsteady. Often the lack of communication skills and confidence further limit your ability to gain access to exercise services.

It all becomes a 'bit too hard' and you tend to STOP exercising, unfortunately making you de-conditioned and unfit. Does this sound familiar?

What we are proposing is a 'shift in thinking' in the physio management of PD and offering help much before the 'traditional physio help' is offered in the under-funded public health system.

---

*What we are proposing is a 'shift in thinking'
in the physio management of PD.*

Now, while all of these aspects of exercise need to be considered in your prescription, the PD Warrior approach can offer you these and so much more. What is unique about PD Warrior is that we have concentrated the patchwork of literature and clinical experience into seven core principles. Lynn's and my interpretation of the literature is that these core principles are the most essential aspects of your exercise program, which is why they underpin the whole philosophy of PD Warrior.

In order to deliver the PD Warrior principles effectively, your instructor needs to be invested in your outcomes and not be your handbrake. The reason I raise this issue is that, time and time again, while teaching PD Warrior to other clinicians, they are stunned to see how hard we push people in PD Warrior. Health concerns aside, PD Warrior is about making change through exercise and it involves challenging, sweat-inducing, muscle-aching hard work. There is no cushioning or hand holding just because you have Parkinson's.

Early days into the creation of PD Warrior, and interested to hear various opinions on what was considered appropriate exercise intensity for people with Parkinson's, I spoke to a well-respected Parkinson's researcher whose reply amazed me. 'I have treated a lot of people with Parkinson's and I have never met anyone who could work that hard.' Not only was I surprised to hear this; I was also incredibly disappointed.

My initial thoughts were that, not only did we have a population of people who were not being treated by tertiary qualified clinicians because their symptoms were considered 'too mild' for therapy (I, too, had been guilty of this), but, when they were treated, they were not being treated effectively. If their therapists didn't think they were capable of working hard enough to receive a training effect and didn't know what to do with them, how would they ever gain enough ground to slow the symptoms of Parkinson's down?

If you are exercising and feel you are working hard, it is likely because you are highly motivated and have found the right person to push you. Pat yourself on the back! Good exercise behaviours are crucial in creating and maintaining long-term control of your condition. However, I can pretty much guarantee that the exercises you are doing, even if strenuous, are still too general and not likely to create the re-wiring in the brain required to help you put your foot down on the gas pedal. If you want to move the best you can and slow the development of your Parkinson's down, general exercise is just not enough.

This needs to change now, for you and for every other person with Parkinson's. This is why I am calling it 'The PD Warrior Revolution'!

Sedentary behaviour

Sedentary behaviour is not a treatment approach, but it deserves a mention here because *it is anti-treatment.*

Sedentary behaviour describes any activity for which energy expenditure is marginally above resting energy levels - that's a nice way of saying you're burning about the same energy as you do when you're asleep. This is best described as being a couch potato - sitting on your butt for prolonged periods, parked in front of your computer, watching TV, or dozing off. How much of your day do you currently spend being sedentary? A sedentary lifestyle is considered to be a major health hazard, leading to increasing rates of Type 2 diabetes, obesity, and cardiovascular disease. There are many reasons why people adopt a sedentary lifestyle. In Parkinson's, these reasons are no different, and unfortunately we can add a few more reasons to the list.

Mood disorders, such as the apathy and depression we discussed in Chapter 1, don't help, as they can suppress motivation to move. Occupations or hobbies that involve prolonged sitting don't help, as they encourage hours expending little energy. Technological advances don't help, as they often eliminate the need to move or apply effort. How much more incidental activity did our grandparents engage in before the invention of the dishwasher, the remote control, the motorcar, and the Internet, to name but a few?

As well as leading to poor general health and premature mortality, it is well known that sedentary behaviours limit physical activity. My personal concern with this is that less physical activity in itself can lead to a self-perpetuating downward spiral of mood changes, loss of fitness, depression, and increasing loss of activity. Coupled with this is the issue of social isolation and lack of participation. There is no doubt that sedentary lifestyles are bad for your health, bad for your mood, and bad for your social life. To hammer home the point even more, adopting a sedentary lifestyle can speed up the development and symptoms of Parkinson's.

Adopting a sedentary lifestyle can speed up the development and symptoms of Parkinson's.

I would encourage you to think about how much activity you typically do at the moment. Activity can be anything from incidental activity, such as doing the housework or walking up to the shops, to concerted physical activity, such as going to the gym. How much do you do? How well are your activities spread across the day? How much time do you spend in a sedentary activity each day?

These are all very important questions to ask yourself and something I will ask you to formalise in Chapter 9, when we discuss the *10-Week Challenge*. PD Warrior is designed to help you get your life back – you will likely do it in 10 weeks, but I want you to learn that PD Warrior is not just about the *10-Week Challenge*; it is about making positive changes for life.

3

The PD Warrior Revolution

'Nothing worthwhile comes easily.'

Nicholas Sparks

The PD Warrior Revolution

It sounds evangelical in a way, but I truly feel like I have 'seen the light'. I believe there is not a single person in the mild stages of idiopathic Parkinson's that PD Warrior will not assist in some way. You are a population who have largely, if inadvertently, been overlooked by health professionals, namely physiotherapists and occupational therapists, because until now we didn't know that there was anything we could do for you in the early stages. This needs to change and it needs to change now.

There is not a single person in the mild stages of idiopathic Parkinson's that PD Warrior will not assist in some way.

PD Warrior is a vehicle of change - change that can help the estimated 50,000 people in the mild to moderate stages of Parkinson's here in Australia and in the rest of the world. My aim is to change the current model of care by delivering exercise as medicine, to deliver

PD Warrior as an early intervention strategy immediately following diagnosis and throughout the course of the disease. My vision is that every single person diagnosed with Parkinson's will be referred straight into PD Warrior as a matter of course - no messing around - as the best early intervention exercise therapy possible.

To do this, I aim to train as many interested health professionals and educate as many individuals with Parkinson's as I possibly can. If you know a health professional working with people with Parkinson's or one who wants to, then PD Warrior is a treatment strategy they cannot afford to overlook.

What exactly is PD Warrior?

PD Warrior is an advanced exercise program that incorporates both physical and cognitive activity for people in the early stages of Parkinson's. PD Warrior has been described as a game changer by neurologists and health professionals because it revolutionises not only the therapy delivered to people newly diagnosed with Parkinson's, but also when it is delivered, how it is delivered, and why it is delivered. The evidence that PD Warrior is based on is already changing the neurological landscape and the way that Parkinson's is managed.

PD Warrior has been described as a game changer by neurologists and health professionals.

At its heart, PD Warrior is an intensive circuit program designed to fight the symptoms of Parkinson's. It is designed specifically to help you in the early stages following diagnosis when your symptoms are still considered mild. PD Warrior is supported by a growing body of evidence that shows that intensive, high-effort, complex exercise has the potential to slow the progression of your symptoms by using neuroplasticity - your brain's natural ability to re-organise its pathways and connections, much like re-wiring. It is this plasticity and capacity for re-wiring that leads to more efficient movement patterns and better motor output. What that means is that, by re-wiring your brain, you can help yourself to move more freely and with less conscious thought. The key to achieving this re-wiring includes being consistent and using the right prescription of exercise.

Unfortunately, over time, the damage to the basal ganglia that is associated with Parkinson's leads to a loss of automatic task generation. Have you ever found yourself walking along while having a conversation, only to stop walking in order to concentrate on continuing your conversation? This is a good example of how an automatic task (walking) has possibly become less automatic with the addition of a second task (talking), thus requiring more conscious attentional processing to continue one or the other.

Most of our everyday movements, such as walking, swallowing, and turning in bed, are beneath conscious thought. You don't normally think about what you are doing - you just do it. With Parkinson's, these movement become less automatic as the damage in the basal ganglia progresses. As your walking becomes less automatic, you are required to consciously think more about your actions. This leaves less attentional capacity to think about other things. It is because of this that dual-task training, performing two tasks simultaneously, is such a big part of PD Warrior. The reality is that you need to be able to do more than one thing at a time in order to function. How many times do you walk and carry the shopping, for instance, or shift the bed sheets while rolling over in bed? That is why we train dual- and multi-tasking. We use any combination of lower limb activity, upper limb activity, and mental processing to challenge you to deal better with the real world.

It is for this reason (as well as others) that PD Warrior is not the same as going to the gym. PD Warrior is an exercise program that is specific to Parkinson's and if you are not doing a similar combination of physical and cognitive exercises, then you may be missing out. Lucky for you, we have done all of the background research and have been tweaking the program since 2012, so your step-by-step home exercise program has already been created for you! One word of caution though: please don't wait until it is too late to make changes.

Don't wait until it is too late to make changes.

Who is PD Warrior for?

PD Warrior will give you the best results if you have recently been diagnosed with idiopathic Parkinson's, are reasonably fit and active, can walk without difficulty through a busy shopping centre, are at low risk of falls, do not have significant issues with freezing, and have no other major health concerns. Think of being able to walk around a busy shopping centre as a proxy for loosely testing your community ambulation, capacity to cope with and negotiate crowded areas, your high-level balance, endurance, and degree of anxiety. If you have stopped doing any of these activities or have begun to find them challenging, you may need further investigation before starting PD Warrior. We have a self-assessment section in Chapter 6 that offers more advice on this. If you can visit a local PD Warrior site, you will be assessed thoroughly prior to entering the PD Warrior program.

PD Warrior circuit classes typically include men and women of all ages and backgrounds. The one thing everyone has in common is their determination to fight the symptoms of Parkinson's. PD Warrior brings together a group of people who no longer feel they are defined by their Parkinson's. To be a PD Warrior, you have to want change and be prepared to work for it. PD Warrior is not for people who think it is a cure or quick fix - it is, instead, a lifestyle choice.

PD Warrior is not for people who think it is a cure or quick fix
- it is, instead, a lifestyle choice.

PD Warrior is suitable for people who have also had neurosurgery, such as DBS (deep brain stimulation). However, it is important that you obtain clearance from your medical team before engaging in any exercise program, especially PD Warrior, when doing this on your own. Everyone with Parkinson's is different and the presentation of symptoms can range in each individual, so we offer many variations of each exercise to help you determine the most suitable level for you. This also applies post-DBS surgery, when the symptoms are likely to be quite different to someone who has not had DBS surgery.

Who is PD Warrior NOT suitable for?

It is important to discuss what persons PD Warrior might *not* be as suitable for. If you are someone who is falling or freezing regularly, has a complex medical history with multiple conditions, has a pre-existing injury, or are recovering from a recent illness, then PD Warrior done in isolation may not be appropriate for you. That doesn't mean that PD Warrior won't help you – in fact, the concepts and philosophy of PD Warrior would almost certainly be beneficial to you – but you would probably benefit more from one-on-one personalised training rather than attempting to start this program alone at home or even attending the circuit style of delivery. Your PD Warrior Instructor will assess you properly and may need to add more mainstream approaches in order to help you out.

If you have any concerns about starting PD Warrior, I strongly encourage you to consult a certified PD Warrior Instructor or, at the very least, your health professional before starting the program.

When should you start PD Warrior?

You should aim to start PD Warrior as soon after diagnosis as possible. If you are already several years post-diagnosis, I encourage you to review Chapter 6 and the self-assessment section carefully to determine whether the program is suitable for you.

Time elapsed since diagnosis is not necessarily indicative of your symptoms or presentation; more likely, your current exercise behaviours and general health will more accurately represent how far your Parkinson's has progressed.

The earlier you start PD Warrior, the more likely you are to see some symptoms and motor problems reverse and your movements improve. I have had clients tell me they are already moving better and feeling more confident in themselves after only an initial assessment and one homework session. I cannot promise the same for you, but isn't it worth a shot?

The milder your symptoms, the easier it is to make those clinical changes. As a general rule, the further along you are, the harder you are going to have to work and the longer you are going to have to stick at it to make smaller gains. But that does not mean that if you were diagnosed years ago, PD Warrior can't help you.

Your success may be defined in different ways. Instead of focusing on purely physical gains, most people further down the line get more out of the psychology of PD Warrior and the ability to improve their sense of self, quality of life, and confidence in movement. Improving your movement, confidence, and overall quality of life is worth the effort. Wouldn't you agree?

The take-home message is that it's never too late to start PD Warrior. Even though it is tailored specifically for people with mild symptoms, you may still benefit from the program when you have more advanced symptoms.

The New Parkinson's Treatment: Exercise is Medicine is designed to furnish you all of the information you need to begin your own PD Warrior program at home. For info on class locations around Australia, visit our website, http://www.pdwarrior.com/locations.

Why should you start PD Warrior?

PD Warrior uses the latest science packaged into an easy to follow program to enable you to get the most out of your exercise program. It differs from mainstream exercise approaches and, for that reason, can be very effective. If you think your symptoms are too mild for the program, you're mistaken! This is precisely the time to get started. There is no such thing as having symptoms too mild to benefit from PD Warrior. What better way to combat your Parkinson's than trying to slow its symptom progression when you are at your most capable!

If you have concluded that you are indeed suitable for the PD Warrior program, congratulations! By taking part in PD Warrior, you are investing in your health and doing everything you can to fight the symptoms of Parkinson's. All you need to do now is read through the rest of the chapters and begin the *10-Week Challenge*. Don't be surprised if you find the exercises more challenging than expected. If they are not difficult to do well, then you are probably not doing them correctly!

How is PD Warrior different to general exercise?

PD Warrior is a series of Parkinson's-specific exercises designed for maximum effect. To finish the *10-Week Challenge*, you should be aiming to achieve the best results for you. As I have said before, it is not the same as other exercise programs, not the same as going to the gym, doing Pilates, or using a personal trainer. If you have been told to keep doing what you were doing before you were diagnosed, then expect little improvement, even if you run marathons. If you want to just keep walking, swimming, or running as you have been doing, expect little neuroplastic change. Exercise of any kind is unquestionably of benefit, but in order to slow the progression of symptoms you're experiencing, the evidence suggests you need to supplement what you're doing with a tailored approach like PD Warrior.

PD Warrior should be challenging, both for your body and mind. The exercises are graded at three levels:

1. Starter – this is where you initiate and get used to an exercise and begin implementing its core principles.
2. Harder – you are familiar with the exercise now and can afford to really work hard at it. Every single repetition counts here.
3. Mental gymnastics – you have mastered the exercise and can increase the complexity by adding a mental task.

If you can do Level 3 without compromising the motor component of the exercise at Level 2, then you have become a black belt PD Warrior! Not many can do this consistently and I look forward to anyone taking up the challenge!

The Evolution of PD Warrior

Back in 2011, having been inspired by attending a radical training program for Parkinson's in the USA, my colleague Lynn Tullock and I began researching the latest international literature and therapy programs for people with Parkinson's. As we looked further into the research, we started to compose a 'shopping list' of goals to incorporate in the design and development of our unique PD Warrior program:

1. Capable of treating all Parkinson's symptoms
2. Can be tailored to each individual
3. Accessible and affordable for large numbers
4. Establishes long-term and positive exercise behaviours
5. Good fun
6. Community-based, not hospital-based
7. Creates a community of like-minded individuals

Lynn and I wanted a model that was diverse enough to treat **all the symptoms of Parkinson's**. We didn't want to target only one symptom, such as slowness of movement or tremor. We wanted a program that could help everyone. PD Warrior is a one size fits all approach in that it may be able to help you regardless of your Parkinson's symptom presentation. If you are tremor-dominant, PD Warrior may help. If you are stiff and rigid, PD Warrior may help. If you have had deep brain stimulation, PD Warrior may help. If your movements are slow and small – you guessed it, PD Warrior may help! Even if you are freezing and falling, PD Warrior may help. I have witnessed this myself.

PD Warrior is a one size fits all approach in that it may help you regardless of your Parkinson's symptom presentation.

We also wanted the program to be specific enough to enable tailoring to each person's individual needs. PD Warrior is not a recipe treatment. There are 10 core exercises that form the base of every home program, but you or your instructor will choose the most appropriate exercises for your situation to best round it out for you. You don't need to do every one of our exercises, and neither are you limited to the 10 core exercises. PD Warrior is a modular program that has more than 150 exercises in its current repertoire. Every single exercise has been created to target a particular symptom, as well as improve your fitness, balance, flexibility, and strength. But, wait, there's more! They're also great fun!

We wanted a program that provides access to a large number of people, ideally outside of the hospital environment. You can do PD Warrior by yourself in your own home with this book (and with our homework helpers: the DVD, app, and webstream circuit classes), one on one with your certified instructor, or as part of a group in the PD Warrior circuit.

One-on-one training with a PD Warrior Instructor really is the most effective delivery for obvious reasons, but, unfortunately, this is not always an option for people for many reasons, usually based around time, money, and other commitments. To get the most out of the PD Warrior circuit or DIY programs, I recommend that every PD Warrior have at least two or three one-on-one sessions with their instructor before entering the circuit to make sure they are well set up with the concepts and technique for their home work. Only then will the PD Warrior circuit be more than sufficient.

The PD Warrior circuit enables larger groups of people to join together and help each other, while also enjoying the expertise of a PD Warrior Instructor at an affordable price. Aside from the cost, group training creates an environment that one-on-one training just cannot provide - an environment of motivation, competition, and fun. If you can get to a local PD Warrior facility, I encourage you to do so. We developed PD Warrior to be delivered in a group because it is an enriched, social environment. This is one of the foundations of PD Warrior and is definitely one of the reasons that it has been so successful. I love watching people leave a PD Warrior circuit class laughing and joking with other PD Warriors they only met an hour earlier.

One of the flaws we saw in most other models was that the programs were delivered in hospitals and they were decidedly NOT fun. PD Warrior is about empowerment – it is not about reinforcing the 'invalid' role that people with Parkinson's can adopt. We try to establish PD Warrior facilities in community settings, such as physiotherapy practices and existing gyms, wherever possible. What we have also tried really hard to do is make PD Warrior fun. It's colourful, engaging, lively, and challenging. The concept is that, if it's fun, you'll keep doing it.

Fundamental Pillars

What sets PD Warrior apart from other programs is its comprehensive philosophy, based on four fundamental pillars:

1. Intensive exercise
2. Life-long behaviour change and adherence to exercise
3. Education and empowerment
4. Support and community

First is the **exercise program** itself. This is the nuts and bolts of the program and where the action happens. It is the exercise program that gives you the courage to fight back by improving your movement. What is unique about our program is the integration of complex physical and cognitive activity, which forces your brain to learn how to move better.

What we feel is even more important than making physical improvements is learning how to maintain those improvements through good **life-long exercise behaviours**. This is the second pillar of PD Warrior and is what may help you to slow the symptoms of Parkinson's down. It's not just about working with you while you are doing the 'formal' part of the program. PD Warrior teaches you how to increase your activity levels, increase your participation in social and domestic tasks, improve your confidence, and get you back into life – and stay there. This is what sets PD Warrior apart and why it has become so successful. Setting you up for good life-long exercise behaviours is the key.

The third pillar of PD Warrior is **education**. You know the old saying: 'With knowledge comes power'. You can turn up and do the exercise and you can increase your activity levels for a short time, but unless you truly understand WHY you are putting all the effort in, you will likely fight a losing battle to maintain your success long term. When you go through the PD Warrior program, you learn things about yourself: what makes you tick, how to motivate yourself, how to keep fighting, and how to get back up and dust yourself off when things get tough. You can do this and feel in control because, with the PD Warrior principles to guide you, you have the education to help yourself.

The final pillar of PD Warrior is **community**. PD Warrior gives you all the tools to cope on your own, but you don't have to fight alone because PD Warrior is working to create a community of like-minded individuals to support you. Even if you are doing the program alone at home, there is always a team of people waiting to help you, support you, and keep you fighting. In this day and age, it doesn't matter where you are - the Internet has brought us closer together than ever before.

I would strongly encourage you to check us out by visiting our Facebook page. Even if you have never used Facebook before, or rarely go online, there has never been a better time to sign up and join the PD Warrior community than right now. Let us help and support you. You don't have to post anything to start with - just read what others have to say and wait until you are ready to post your first success!

Important things to keep in mind when doing PD Warrior

1. The companion website

The website is a very useful tool that can support you in your PD Warrior *10-Week Challenge*. The website offers a range of support services designed to assist you at every step of the way and it links you in to a community of people who are just like you – motivated to get back into life. You will find videos of the core PD Warrior exercises as well as a range of new exercises that you can add to your program. On the *10-Week Challenge* page, you can register for your *10-Week Challenge*. You will get weekly emails, including your assessment pack and tips and advice to keep you motivated. You can even participate in live PD Warrior circuit classes through our webstream. Find other products, like our DVD and Home Starter Kit, that make starting and sticking with PD Warrior even easier.

Visit the website here: http://www.pdwarrior.com.

2. Facebook

PD Warrior has its own Facebook page, which is a meeting place where you can make friends, become inspired, and provide your own comments and thoughts. Please visit the PD Warrior Facebook page at http://www.facebook/pdwarriorprogram.

3. Complete your self-assessment

The self-assessment section of the book is your opportunity to obtain baseline measures for yourself before you start PD Warrior, which you can compare to where you are after you've completed our *10-Week Challenge*. The idea is to do the self-assessment tests before you start the *10-Week Challenge* and then again shortly after you finish. You should not assess or compare your results within those ten weeks of the Challenge or it will introduce bias when you come to do your post-test scores. (We will explore this in greater detail in Chapter 6.)

There are four tests in the self-assessment section: a quality of life questionnaire, one that measures functional capacity, another is a fitness test, and the final test is a balance test. The self-assessment should not take you too long to do - give yourself at least 30 minutes to complete the self-assessment section.

4. **Record your efforts**

I cannot emphasise enough how important it is to record your efforts during the *10-Week Challenge*. Recording your sessions and the effort levels achieved are really important to keep you motivated throughout the *10-Week Challenge*.

I would also encourage you to chart your progress. To do this, you need to have a longer-term goal that you are working towards, and perhaps some smaller goals to achieve along the way. Charting your progress can help to drive you towards your big goal. Achieving your goal can be one of the most rewarding moments of the program. Don't worry if you can't think of a goal at this moment. There is a whole section on goal planning in Chapter 8 to help you. The most important thing for you to focus on at the moment is the commitment you are making to yourself, to your family, and to your other loved ones to start fighting the symptoms of Parkinson's.

5. **Involve your family and friends**

Please do not make the mistake of trying to do PD Warrior on your own. The PD Warrior *10-Week Challenge* is designed to be challenging. If it is not, then you are probably not doing it correctly. Set yourself up for success by enlisting family members to support you by buddying up. At our PD Warrior sites, we encourage you to bring a buddy to the classes free of charge for this very reason. An objective third party involved in your program will double your chances of success and provide further reinforcement and motivation when you're working from home.

The role of your buddy is explained further in Chapters 6 and 8 but, put simply, your buddy is there to help pull you through the tough days and lift you even higher on your good days. Choose your buddy wisely. Your buddy needs to be someone positive and encouraging and also someone you respect and trust, because you will need to listen to them and often follow their direction, even if you disagree.

4

PD Warrior Principles

'With knowledge comes power.'
Meiji Stewart

PD Warrior is structured around a framework of seven core principles and in this combination of principles lies the power of PD Warrior. When we talk about driving neuroplasticity, what we are really talking about is creating an exercise environment in which you are challenging your brain to learn and become more efficient. These seven core principles create the specific environment to promote neuroplasticity and create long-term improvements that may help to slow the progression of symptoms down.

Since 2011, Lynn and I have been researching the literature, comparing existing exercise programs for people with and without Parkinson's, and testing different strategies ourselves. We have distilled our extensive knowledge of the literature and what is currently available into the PD Warrior Seven Core Principles.

It is critical to know *how* to apply the seven core principles of PD Warrior in order to achieve the best results, so let's take a moment to take a closer look.

Understanding the principles and being able to apply them appropriately will enable you to get the most out of your DIY, circuit, or one-on-one sessions. All of our PD Warrior Instructors are highly trained to recognise what your main problems are so that they can tailor each of the circuit stations especially for you. But it's not enough for them to understand the underlying principles – you need to grasp them too, so nothing is left to chance.

The seven core PD Warrior principles are:

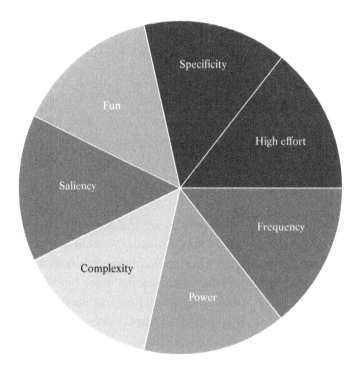

1. Specificity

The first core principle is Specificity. This relates to the ability of the PD Warrior program to target your specific needs directly. Your needs are unique to you. Everyone with Parkinson's presents slightly differently, so you should not assume that you should be doing your exercises the same way as your neighbour. Some people are troubled more with tremors and others with slowness of movement or dyskinesias. Some may be struggling more with mood disturbances and anxiety. What are your greatest challenges with regard to your Parkinson's? Your activity limitations and what you are struggling with will shape the exercises most appropriate to you.

Everyone does not follow the same treatment recipe. It's not about adding five reps of this and ten reps of that to mimic everyone else. Each exercise you do is tailored to the challenges you face to make it harder or easier. You may have one main problem, or several that require a specific individual approach. Depending on the problem(s), there is a practical application of specificity. For example:

- If your main problem is tremor, you may find it helpful to focus on more of the forced-use components of the program, such as sprint training on a bike, treadmill, or power-walking around the block.
- If your primary struggle is with bradykinesia, you may find it helpful to focus on more of the amplitude-based training.
- If anxiety is paramount, you may find it helpful to focus on the education and self-empowerment part of the program.
- If you find coordination of multiple tasks difficult, you may find it helpful to add more dual-tasking complexity early on in the program.

Each exercise you do is tailored to the challenges you face.

Specificity is important when considering your goals as well as your exercises. What precisely do you want to achieve by doing PD Warrior? Do you want to get better at doing up buttons or turning the pages of a book? Do you want to be able to walk down the street with more confidence? Your goals are important and need to be included in the planning of your PD Warrior program to help tailor it to you specifically.

The PD Warrior motto is 'no challenge, no change'. This is what sets PD Warrior apart from other treatment approaches. Traditional therapy focuses on the 'Use it or lose it' principle. If you are sedentary and deconditioned, you will lose mobility, and not just because of your Parkinson's.

PD Warrior is different because not only has it been designed to help you slow the deterioration of your Parkinson's down, but it has also been designed to help you improve your symptoms in the early stages so that you may move more freely and feel more in control.

Write down what you consider to be your top three biggest problems. Are they tremor, slow movement, or anxiety for instance? Do you need to work more on your upper limbs, legs, or balance? This will jumpstart you into thinking about how you can best design your DIY program.

2. **High effort**

The second core principle is effort level. High effort means what it says: your exercise program needs to be effortful, strenuous, and should challenge you every time. I am going to say that again – it should challenge you *every time!* In PD Warrior, there are no points for simply turning up and going through the motions. Not only do you have to be present, but you also have to be committed to working hard. Traditional therapy approaches do not work people hard enough, and certainly, in my experience, do not push people much past their self-selected pace.

In PD Warrior, there are no points for simply turning up and going through the motions.

What is self-selected pace? This is the rate that you choose to work at voluntarily, the degree of effort you choose to expend. It's the rate that 80 per cent of people at the gym work at while on the treadmill or exercise bike. You know – the rate that you can still exercise at, yet drift off and think about other things or watch TV. Self-selected pace is the rate that holds you back from possibly improving your symptom presentation. It is not your fault. People tend to work at a rate comfortable for them. It doesn't matter whether they are going for a jog, swim, or walk around the block. Left to their own devices, most people will work at a steady but *comfortable* pace. Evidence tells us that if you do these exercises at self-selected pace, you are unlikely to see improvements beyond your general fitness.

Now, let's clarify what high effort means and, as important, what it does not mean. High effort does not mean high impact or high intensity. These are three different things.

High impact is exercise that is focused on creating high levels of gravitational force to the body and is most commonly seen with jumping, hopping, and leaping activities that require you to be airborne for a short period of time. Some advanced levels of certain PD Warrior exercises are classified as high impact; however, this is not the emphasis of PD Warrior exercises and you should only be doing these exercise levels if appropriate for you and your particular program.

High intensity is exercise that is focused on high-level cardiovascular fitness training or high-intensity resistance training. Exercises that you may commonly associate with high-intensity training include running, step-ups, and boxing. PD Warrior certainly can give you a good cardiovascular workout and you will inevitably be fitter and stronger when you finish the program, but its emphasis is not on high intensity.

High effort in PD Warrior consists of exercise that generates a high motor output. What is motor output? This is your ability to drive movement that is powerful, crisp, and strong, movement quality that is the opposite to the symptoms of Parkinson's. All of the movements you do in PD Warrior should feel vigorous and require a lot of energy for you to complete them. Remember, just going through the motions will not get you over the line. If you want to be a PD Warrior, you have to fight your symptoms like a PD Warrior. Once you start to appreciate the level of effort required to move like a PD Warrior, you will not look back.

It can be difficult to gauge your effort levels initially, especially if you are not used to working hard. There are several scales that can be used to rate your perceived exertion (RPE). I have taken the liberty of modifying a commonly used RPE scale to make it easier to apply to PD Warrior. This scale is a self-recorded percentage measure of effort. Take a look at it here and, when you are doing your PD Warrior program, remember that your RPE goal is 80 per cent!

PD Warrior: Rate of Perceived Exertion (RPE) Scale

10%	I'm not even pretending to do this exercise.
20%	I'm doing the exercise with insignificant effort.
30%	I'm going through the motions and feel less than impressive.
40%	I could do this exercise all day.
50%	I could do this exercise at least fifty times and not break a sweat.
60%	I am starting to generate power and force in my movements.
70%	I am starting to feel athletic and definitely breaking a sweat.
80%	**I am powerful and feisty – I am moving like a PD Warrior!**
90%	I risk levitating because I am moving so vigorously.
100%	I'm going to hurt myself, someone next to me, or the furniture.

You should aim to build up to an effort level in the target zone of 80 per cent in all of your movements. If you rate yourself at 40 per cent, you might as well just thank yourself for turning up and then pack up and finish. If you rate yourself at 60 per cent, you should be starting to feel like you are moving remarkably well. I find that 60 per cent RPE is often a plateau, a sticking point for many people, and it can take a few sessions before people can push through to 70 and 80 per cent.

The hardest part of using an RPE is learning how to rate yourself independently. You may be used to moving at abnormally low effort levels if your movements have become smaller and slower over time. Use the playback on your video camera and grab your buddy to improve the disconnect between the effort level you might be feeling with the effort level the rest of the world might be seeing.

Either way, using an RPE scale is not easy unless you are taught how to use it well. The ideal way to learn how to use it correctly is with a PD Warrior Instructor. Even if you can only get yourself to a PD Warrior location for a single session, it can mean the difference between achieving average versus spectacular results. If you just cannot get to a PD Warrior facility, then you can hop on the website in the How to Get Started section (www.pdwarrior.com.how-to-get-started).

Working at high effort is a core principle of PD Warrior, so remember to use the RPE and rate yourself every time you do your PD Warrior program and any incidental activity.

3. Frequency

Frequency is absolutely essential to drive the neuroplastic changes in your brain and develop the necessary skill to move at a higher effort level consistently. If you do PD Warrior once a week, you might get fitter, stronger, or move better, but it is not guaranteed. If you do PD Warrior twice a week, you will likely start to make small gains. If you commit to doing PD Warrior every day during the *10-Week Challenge*, you give yourself the best chance to not only impress yourself but to impress your family and those around you.

Doing PD Warrior every day during the *10-Week Challenge* will give you the best chance of success.

Frequency is important because your brain responds to the demands you place on it. If you do a task more frequently, you reinforce the circuits and pathways in your brain associated with that task. Over time, the movements that drive that task become more efficient, more automatic, and use less conscious brainpower. Remember that your brain is not capable of consciously focusing on every single movement you do during the day. We would literally struggle to get out of bed in the morning if there were no circuits and pathways in our brains that 'knew' how to get us out of bed automatically.

You can train yourself to do more things at the same time. However, in order for this to become meaningful and relevant in everyday life, you need to practice it frequently and in a variety of different settings. It is well known that Olympic athletes complete thousands of repetitions over hundreds of hours of training to get better. Your *10-Week Challenge* is going to be the same. You will be expected to train twice every single day during the program. If you are attending a PD Warrior facility on select days, you only need to train once more that day. If you are completely DIY, then you will need to do your exercises twice a day. Every day.

If you want to change your life, you need to commit. Aim for at least 20 minutes of PD Warrior exercise twice a day during the *10-Week Challenge*. If you are not consistent and frequent, you will be disappointed.

Frequency is the third core principle of PD Warrior because we want the best results for you, not just in the *10-Week Challenge* but for life!

4. Power

Have you noticed that you feel 'weaker' because of your Parkinson's? There is evidence that weakness is a primary impairment of Parkinson's. There is no doubt that people with Parkinson's tend to be weaker, especially in the limb where Parkinson's first emerged.

Current thinking about the cause of this weakness suggests that it is a signalling problem from your brain to the muscles. A weak signal inhibits efficient recruitment and speed of muscle contraction. It is believed that Parkinson's doesn't affect the muscles directly, but, over time, the muscle starts to atrophy and deteriorate because it is not getting used to its full potential.

The philosophy behind power training is to emphasise strength and amplitude in your movements, to teach you how to recruit and contract your muscles as efficiently as you can.

Strength training in PD Warrior is about pushing through the barrier that hinders your motor output and makes your movements slow and small. It is about accessing your ability to generate high-effort movement and effectively contract your muscles when required, for every movement, not just the PD Warrior exercises.

Amplitude training is making sure that you achieve the full, perhaps even exaggerated, range of available movement possible. Training in this way is designed to offset the inherent inclination to be small.

In order to be powerful, you need to incorporate both amplitude and strength training to help you combat the weakness and the small, slow movements that often drive your patience to the limits.

Try this activity now. Clench your fist and open it again fast. Repeat this several times. Are you stretching your fingers apart and straight each time you open your hand? Are they extended and strong or are they curved and soft? What about your wrist? Are you getting a stretch at the front of your wrist as well? It is very common to develop shortening of the soft tissue in your hand and wrist over time because you don't consistently use the full range of movement available to you.

Your movements have likely become under-scaled in both amplitude and strength. You have lost your power. Because it has happened gradually, your slow, small movements have become 'normal' to you. Your scale of strength and amplitude has been re-calibrated. For this reason, power training is important if your movements are slow and small.

It is not enough to just do bigger, stronger movements during PD Warrior though - it needs to become part of everything you do. With all of the core principles of PD Warrior, it is not about performance on the day, in the gym, or in front of your instructor. The whole program is designed to make long-lasting change to movement in ALL of the tasks you do during any given day.

PD Warrior is designed to make long-lasting change to movement in ALL of the tasks you do during any given day.

A good way to start introducing power training into your day, apart from the PD Warrior exercises, is to swing your arms in a power march the next time you go for a walk. Be powerful and make sure your arm swing and stride length are slightly exaggerated. Do not be surprised if you feel ridiculous and self-conscious! If your movements have re-calibrated to be small and slow, and they probably have, even in the early stages of Parkinson's, then this will feel very strange. Then, ask your buddy what you look like doing this. They will probably report that you look powerful and confident, perhaps even better than you have looked in some time. If you are not convinced, take a video of yourself power walking.

Power training is most effective in people who complain of weakness as well as slow and small movements. It is rare that I recommend power training in isolation, but there is no question that it plays a large role in the program and why it is one of the core principles of PD Warrior.

5. Complexity

Ideally, by now you have a better understanding of some of the crucial elements in doing PD Warrior and why it is so important that you do your program regularly and frequently. However, repetition alone does not drive the skill acquisition and the motor learning necessary to create lasting change and regain some of the automaticity of your movements. There is a little more to it than this, which is why complexity is the fifth core principle.

In order for your brain to learn, you need to not only be teaching it frequently, but also challenging it to problem solve each time. This involves greater complexity than repetition alone. It is the complexity of the exercise that enables greater generalisation to everyday tasks. All of the PD Warrior exercises you do will be based on a daily task that most people with Parkinson's have difficulty doing. The beauty of the PD Warrior exercises is that, because they are based on everyday tasks, by adding an additional layer of difficulty, the exercises may help to improve your overall capacity to do more than one thing at a time in everyday life.

There are many ways in which complexity can be added to the PD Warrior exercises. One of the most obvious ways is to ensure there is an element of timing. Many people with Parkinson's have difficulty keeping time to a beat, especially when a weight shift from one leg to the other is required and if the beat is quite fast. Metronomes have long been used in traditional physiotherapy as an auditory cue to facilitate stepping when you freeze. I like to use a metronome in many of the PD Warrior exercises, not as a cue but to challenge timing. You do not need to use a metronome. Another easy way to challenge timing is by moving to a good tune with a strong beat. For walking, you can start with a song that has about 80 beats per minute. (Certain music collections targeted for exercise list the beats per minute of each song. You may also find this information online.) Try stepping to the beat consistently. A great side benefit of a good song is that it can put a smile on your face while you exercise, especially if it is one you really like.

Another obvious way to add complexity to a PD Warrior exercise is to have your arms and legs do separate tasks. Just as rubbing your tummy and patting your head involves a high degree of attentional focus and complexity, so, too, can doing different, simultaneous exercises with your arms and legs. Many of the PD Warrior exercises have a basic level of complexity involving tasks with just your legs. Once you have mastered the timing and motor skill of the task in the legs, we ask you to engage the arms and hands in a different task, while keeping to the same beat. It is important when adding the hands and arms to an exercise that you do not compromise the timing and power of the legs. This is often where people become unstuck and start to think an exercise is easy.

As you become more competent with the exercise, added layers of difficulty can be introduced by changing the environment, introducing a mental task to be completed at the same time, or changing the focus of your attention. In my clinic, we typically use an MP3 player that has pre-recorded cognitive tasks on it in order to add complexity. You can download this dual-tasking track for use at home when you reach this level. To get the dual-tasking track, visit our website's 'How to Get Started' page, http://www.pdwarrior.com/how-to-get-started.

One of the key elements to note about introducing complexity to a task is that a PD Warrior exercise should never be easy for you to do. It should be physically and mentally demanding. If it feels easy, then you are not adding enough power and likely not enough complexity. Your brain will certainly not be learning anything new. It is a fine balance and may take some time to get used to. Think of the Goldilocks Principle: it shouldn't be so hard that you fall apart trying to add too many components together, and it shouldn't be so easy that there is no challenge. The exercise should be 'ju-u-u-ust right'. It should be an *achievable* challenge for you, through concentration and effort.

Complexity is one of the best ways to make your program more relevant to your day-to-day life and is a great way to challenge you with even the most straightforward motor tasks. Complexity is one of my favourite core principles of PD Warrior.

PD Warrior exercises should
never be easy to do.

---

6. Saliency

Your PD Warrior program needs to be salient and meaningful to you and your therapy goals. There are several reasons why this is important and not least of all because, generally, people only like to put effort into things that are important to them. If you do not value the PD Warrior program and the potential benefits that it will bring you, then you are less likely to schedule your exercise as a priority. PD Warrior needs to resonate with you. Vague goals, such as 'I want to move better', will not be specific enough to really drive you forward, especially on the days when you find exercising tough.

One of the best ways for you to be successful with PD Warrior is to isolate what is most meaningful to you and what benefits you want to get in return for your investment in time and energy. In Chapter 8, you will consider ways to increase your intrinsic motivation, set your goals, and identify barriers that might prevent success. First, let's take a look at what is most salient to you by examining what you want to achieve in PD Warrior a bit more closely. A good example of this might be:

I need to exercise because I want to move better.

Now, think about why that is important to you, and add that:

I want to move better because I want to be able to keep up with my friends when we all go walking.

At a deeper level, perhaps you might write:

I feel embarrassed when my friends have to wait for me to catch up.

Can you dig even more deeply? Why is that important to you?

Because my friends are important to me and I do not want them to pity me or give up on me.

You are now not just exercising for your body but also for your social life and your self-esteem. That has a lot more meaning than simply stating, 'I want to move better'.

That particular scenario may not apply to you, but the concept is the same. You need to find a way to make your exercise relevant. Come up with as many meaningful statements as you can. Use these as your anchor points and they will become the reasons why you are motivated to exercise.

PD Warrior makes your exercise
relevant and meaningful to you.

---

7. **Fun!**

One of the most important things about PD Warrior is how much fun it is. Yes, it is exercise and, yes, it needs to be hard work to be effective, but the program is set up to be fun, engaging, and keep you interested in your progress and that of the others around you.

We strive to keep re-inventing the program so that it is fresh, novel, challenging, and inspiring. We search out interesting equipment to use, great music, and functional exercises. We consistently encourage PD Warriors to give us feedback on what they like and don't like.

> PD Warrior is designed to be fun, engaging,
> and keep you interested in your progress.

Most of our PD Warriors comment on the spirit of camaraderie that develops through the program. Although you may not be able to make it to a PD Warrior circuit, using tools like the PD Warrior Facebook page can be a great way to receive the help and advice that you need. Remember, a PD Warrior need never train alone.

PD Warrior should be fun for you at home too. If you haven't already looked at the support products, such as the DVD, app, and webstream, check them out. They can help keep PD Warrior fun. Every now and then, consider re-reading Chapter 8 for a recap on how to maintain your motivation level.

5

Things to Consider before Doing PD Warrior

'Every man dies, but not every man lives.'

Garth Brooks

PD Warrior was designed to give everyone with early-stage Parkinson's access to the right type of exercise to help slow the symptoms of Parkinson's down. This illustrated book supports you to do this from your own living room as part of your own DIY PD Warrior program. It is not designed to replace the expertise of, or the face-to-face sessions with, a PD Warrior Instructor but, rather, to give you the opportunity to access the right exercise if you can't get to a PD Warrior location.

Consult your PD Warrior Instructor or health professional

Booking in for an assessment with a PD Warrior Instructor can go a long way to helping you get the most out of your program and avoiding any adverse events. For information on class locations around Australia, visit our website, http://www.pdwarrior.com/locations.

PD Warrior is best started as soon after diagnosis as possible. Exercise is good for the brain and there is the suggestion that it can even protect your neurons from further destruction. If you have been recently diagnosed, it can be tough coming to terms with your diagnosis. This is normal and many people really benefit from the supportive and inspiring environment the PD Warrior community creates. We won't necessarily offer to hold your hand, but we will ask if you are ready to fight. When you feel ready, start by doing something positive for yourself and contact the closest PD Warrior Instructor and join the Facebook community.

Most people go one of two ways when they are diagnosed with Parkinson's. They are either eager to start an exercise program, but are often not sure what the best program is, or they want nothing more than to go to bed, crawl into a ball, and give up. If you have bought this book, then I'm guessing you are a member of the first group and want to play an active role in your treatment. If you feel more like those in the second group, and perhaps someone who loves you has given you this book, I want to encourage you to take that positive first step towards improving your quality of life by starting to exercise and joining the PD Warrior revolution. You're not alone.

If you are doing PD Warrior from this book without first seeing a PD Warrior Instructor, then I recommend that you at least consult a health professional before starting the program to make sure you are fit enough to start safely and have no pre-existing injuries that you are going to aggravate. If you hurt yourself or exacerbate an underlying issue, you are unlikely to get the results you are looking for and end up feeling disappointed. It is always a good idea to get yourself checked over before starting any new exercise program, especially one this intense.

Pre-existing injury

If you have a pre-existing injury, then you really need to consider whether you are sufficiently fit to participate in PD Warrior. There is no point in flaring up or worsening an existing injury. If you suffer from a musculoskeletal injury or condition other than Parkinson's, or develop any problems during the program, please immediately seek advice from your health professional prior to continuing. Many of the exercises can be easily modified to minimise the impact on certain body parts but you may need a little help with this.

How do I avoid injuring myself?

It is important that you carefully follow the instructions for each exercise to avoid injury. If you are just starting out, go easy, especially if you are new to exercise or haven't exercised regularly. As you become more confident with the program and the exercises themselves, you can start to work towards the target effort level of 80 per cent. It is normal to feel a certain amount of muscle strain and soreness in the days following PD Warrior, especially when they are novel exercises and your muscles are not used to them, but if anything hurts while you are doing PD Warrior, stop immediately. Again, all of the exercises can be modified to be made easier (as well as harder), so listen to your body for cues.

Common areas of injury, if you use poor technique or over-exert yourself, are the shoulders and lower back. These areas can really give you grief if you have a history of problems in these areas, are stiff or weak, and start loading up before you are ready.

Shoulder pain

Not long ago, I informally surveyed 31 members of the community that we treat with Parkinson's in the Advance Rehab Centre gym. Now, although my survey wouldn't stand up to any rigorous peer review, it was helpful to learn that the most common pre-existing complaints these people mentioned were shoulder pain (78%) and poor posture (63%). Approximately 10 per cent of the general adult population are reported to experience an episode of shoulder pain in their lifetime. Either we have a really unlucky population of people, or I might be on to something here. Do you have a problem with your shoulders? Pain or stiffness that limits some of your activities? If so, you might be surprised to hear that PD Warrior generally helps most cases of shoulder pain.

My theory is – and I am not a shoulder expert by any means – that general stiffness and poverty of movement (commonly seen as loss of arm swing when walking) leads to learned non-use, immobility weakness, loss of coordination of the rotator cuff muscles, and secondary stiffness at the level of the soft tissue itself. All of this commonly leads to shoulder dysfunction, pain, and loss of movement. PD Warrior may help to break this cycle by encouraging greater range of motion, greater recruitment of muscles, and increased overall use of the shoulder. This, in time, improves general strength, rotator cuff coordination, and reduces stiffness in the shoulder.

A word of caution: not everyone experiences this improvement, especially when there is significant underlying shoulder pathology, such as a torn rotator cuff muscle, arthritic and degenerative changes, or an irritation of the bursa or tendons. It is important, if you have a problem with your shoulders, to have it looked at by someone who 'knows their stuff' about shoulders. I would recommend seeing an experienced physiotherapist who works in the musculoskeletal area first. If you do have a shoulder pathology, follow the advice of your physiotherapist and modify the PD Warrior program as recommended, so that you do not exacerbate any injuries.

Shoulder problems can be inherently tricky to manage, and all of that talk on shoulders doesn't even start to account for the change in posture adopted by many with Parkinson's. Changes in your posture can also lead to long-term shoulder dysfunction, as the shoulder blade no longer maintains the right rhythm with the upper arm. The take-home message is that your shoulder pain may not be an isolated shoulder problem and you probably should have it looked at before you start PD Warrior.

Poor posture

Thoracic stiffness and stooping can be a direct result of rigidity in the trunk. It is not uncommon to see someone with very early Parkinson's who has lost flexibility and movement in the spine, especially rotation. Walking with this loss of axial rotation and rigid trunk movement looks like walking with a plywood board strapped to your back – no movement of the arms and shoulders and no rotation of the trunk over the pelvis as you step. Is this you?

Do you look like you have the weight of the world on your shoulders? Is your head tipped forwards, pushing you into a stooped position?

Poor posture is very common in those with Parkinson's. There are many neurological and musculoskeletal reasons why this can occur. Few of them are inevitable. Apart from the aesthetics of poor posture (which is what most people complain to me about), a stooping posture can negatively affect your breathing. The stiffness of the bony thoracic cage and reduced mechanical area to fill your lungs can also be associated with rigidity of your thoracic muscles, all which can make breathing more difficult. If you are reasonably fit and mobile now, you may not notice this, but if you let your fitness slide and become increasingly more deconditioned, the increasing demand for oxygen during daily exertion may make any difficulty with breathing more apparent.

Poor posture is very common in those with Parkinson's. There are many neurological and musculoskeletal reasons why this can occur. Few are inevitable.

Falls

Have you had a fall in the past twelve months? If so, one of the biggest risk factors you face is having another fall. As Parkinson's progresses, falls can become a serious problem, leading to injury, loss of confidence, decreasing mobility, and social isolation. There are some staggering statistics from the literature stating that up to 70 per cent of people with Parkinson's fall each year, and about half of those will fall more than once. Up to 90 per cent of people with Parkinson's fall at home, mostly when standing, walking, or turning. Falling as a consequence of having Parkinson's typically indicates that you have lost your postural stability. This usually occurs at the moderate stages of Parkinson's, although around a third of people with Parkinson's will have a problem with their balance within two years of diagnosis.

At the moment, there is little evidence to show that once you start having falls, you can improve the situation significantly. Most of the interventions in these studies are exercise programs based on strength and balance training. This is logical when you think that strength and balance correlate highly and it is a loss of balance that often leads to falls. What most of the interventions lack though are most of the principles on which PD Warrior is based. That is large-amplitude, powerful movement training combined with high-effort, frequent, complex dual-tasking exercises. We have yet to research falls prevention in our PD Warrior population, so I can only comment from my clinical experience, but this is what my gut tells me: falls are best prevented in the first place with a multipart exercise program, such as PD Warrior, that is designed specifically for the impairments seen in Parkinson's. However, if you are falling already, don't believe that all is lost. Exercise of the intensity of PD Warrior, in my experience, has reduced the number of falls in many of our patients.

A quick caveat: PD Warrior was not designed for people who are already falling. PD Warrior often involves challenging physical and mental activity that may put you at risk of further falls. The last thing I want is for you to fall while doing PD Warrior at home. If you are falling, it doesn't mean that you can't participate in PD Warrior; it just means that you need to be careful when doing the program. There are notes in the exercise section on how to modify the exercises if you are someone who is already at risk of falling. If you have any doubts about any of the exercises and your capacity to do them safely, please avoid them until you talk to your health professional. It is better to be careful than overconfident in your balance when starting out and to follow the instructions carefully, especially if you are exercising on your own.

As a side note, it is always a good idea to clear your workout area of any sharp-edged furniture, mats, glass, loose cables, and anything else that might cause you to trip or suffer injury.

Freezing

Freezing is characterised by an inability to initiate a movement or becoming frozen in the middle of a movement. Many people will describe freezing when walking as suddenly having glue stuck to their feet. Typical areas that people will report freezing are changes in flooring such as when going from kitchen tiles to lounge room carpet, turning tight corners, and negotiating furniture, sometimes even when there is a clear level surface but you grind to a halt. Freezing, combined with the smaller, shuffling gait patterns often seen in later stages of Parkinson's, can present a huge risk for falls. Understandably, if your feet tend to end up close together instead of slightly spread apart, you will have a narrower base of support, which can become a problem in turning and reaching past your centre of gravity.

PD Warrior is not designed specifically to assist with the problems of freezing. Generally, if people report episodes of freezing during the assessment, we screen them carefully to make sure that they are safe to come into a PD Warrior circuit. Occasionally, some people may not be ready initially but, following a few individual sessions, we develop effective strategies for them to deal with their freezing so that they can more safely participate in the PD Warrior circuit.

If you experience episodes of freezing, please consider whether PD Warrior is appropriate for you and, if so, time your exercise when you are at your best and 'on' your medication.

The importance of following instructions

If you have decided to do PD Warrior in isolation, without attending a PD Warrior facility for assessment or exercise instruction, it is extremely important that you take the time to read this book thoughtfully, from front to back, and register for the *10-Week Challenge* on the website before attempting any of the PD Warrior activities. Complete the self-assessment section carefully first, and be realistic about whether PD Warrior is appropriate for you.

When you start the program, follow the instructions, especially the modifications on how to make each exercise harder or easier, depending on your level. While it is important to work hard on each exercise, and exert yourself, don't overdo it. You will get a lot more out of the program if you work at the appropriate level for you (which is why an assessment or one or more individual training sessions are so beneficial.) Falling over, injuring yourself, or losing interest because you have pitched the exercises at too difficult a level for you will not give you the results you want.

If you have any further questions, the website, http://www.pdwarrior.com is a great resource to help you.

6

How to Get Started

The secret to getting ahead is getting started.

By now, I hope that you are getting excited about the possibilities open to you through PD Warrior. If you exercise regularly, you will already be familiar with some of the information in this chapter. You should expect to come out of the *10-Week Challenge* in peak physical and mental condition.

You should expect to come out of the *10-Week Challenge* in peak physical and mental condition.

In order to really get the most out of PD Warrior, you will need to set some objective measures. Objective measures are useful tools to help you to establish a baseline (your starting point) and track your improvements over time. This is essential because you need to be able to grade yourself and choose the appropriate complexity level of each PD Warrior exercise at the start and then compare your initial outcomes with your results at the end of your *10-Week Challenge* to see how far you've come.

If you are committed to doing the 10-Week Challenge, I encourage you to post your goals on the PD Warrior Facebook page. As I

57

mentioned before, this kind of public statement that you are ready to join the PD Warrior revolution will help to keep you accountable and help others to support you in your goals. PD Warrior is a community and I invite you to become part of it by dropping by the Facebook page to say hello and be inspired by what other participants have to say.

How to perform the self-assessment measures

Self-assessment can be an effective way to gauge your pre- and post-measure scores, however, they can also be plagued with bias. Bias is introduced when you expect to achieve a certain outcome and re-test yourself against the expected scores. Most people in this instance are likely to over-estimate their scores for a positive effect. It is really important when completing these questionnaires that you be as honest as you can. Be brutal. These results are not for anyone else but you. In some of the questionnaires, such as the PDQ-8, you will be asked not to overthink your answers and tick the first response that comes to mind. In other questionnaires, such as the SPDDS, you will be asked to take a little more time answering the questions to make sure you have explored all scenarios. I have not made up any of these tools; they are all standard measures used and tested by health professionals around the world, and to them I am thankful, as it helps us to all speak a common language! The PDQ-8 Questionnaire, in particular, is provided solely for personal use by people with Parkinson's for illustrative informational purposes only, under licence from the licensor (Isis Innovation Limited), and no reliance on, commercial use, or reproduction may be made of the questionnaire from the publication without the user first obtaining a licence to do so from the licensor.

Start by signing up to the PD Warrior *10-Week Challenge* by entering your email here: http://pdwarrior.com/10-week-challenge. The *10-Week Challenge* is one of the best ways to help keep you motivated. Not only does it give you an end point and something to work towards, but you can also align your short-term goals to the *10-Week Challenge.*

Once you have signed up, you will receive an email each week designed to help keep you on track. Week One is about getting you organised. You will be emailed a copy of the self-assessment sheets. Please download and print them out and start working your way through them.

On the PD Warrior Facebook page you can meet someone else who may be starting the challenge at the same time as you are. Our Facebook page is a great place to share your thoughts as you move through the program together.

All of these strategies are designed to help you stay motivated in the early stages.

If you give the *10-Week Challenge* a really good go, our research shows that you are more likely to adopt good exercise behaviours and continue with exercise after the *10-Week Challenge* finishes. For more information on the *10-Week Challenge,* read Chapter 9 and visit our website.

If you have registered on the website for the *10-Week Challenge*, you will have received the following test papers by email now, (you will also find these in the back of the book, from page 155);

1. PDQ-8
2. Self-Assessment PD Disability Scale (SPDDS)
3. 6-minute walk test
4. Berg Balance Score

Remember, doing the self-assessment is not a race. Once you have performed all the tests and recorded your measures, pop them in a folder or tuck them into the back of this book. *Do not look at them again until after you have completed your 10-Week Challenge and retaken the self-assessment.* Only then should you compare them with your current post-challenge results.

1. PDQ-8

The PDQ-8 has eight questions relating to mobility, daily living activities, emotional wellbeing, social support, cognition, communication, and bodily discomfort, that is, your overall quality of life as it relates to your Parkinson's. Before starting any part of the program, please answer this questionnaire while reflecting over the previous month.

When you have finished, total your scores into one grand total – the single index. The scoring is pretty straight forward;

0 = never
1 = occasionally
2 = sometimes
3 = often
4 = always/unable

The highest possible score is 32 while the lowest score is 0. Divide your grand total by 32 and multiply by 100 to get your final score.

Formula for the PDQ-8 Single Index

$$\frac{\text{sum of scores of each question}}{32} \times 100$$

The lower your final score, the better. However, while it is important to know where you sit on the continuum, what is more important is how you compare to yourself along your journey. When it comes time to re-test yourself, we will talk about how to compare the results.

2. Self-Assessment PD Disability Scale (SPDDS)

This form asks you to consider how difficult it is for you to complete certain set tasks. It gives you a single score that can be standardised before and after your *10-Week Challenge*. I find that sometimes my clients have not thought about questions like this before, and answer too quickly that they can do all tasks without difficulty. It is only with further probing that I discover any number of activity modifications or difficulties that have been subconsciously swept under the carpet.

Take your time answering this questionnaire and really think about the last few times you completed each task. Have you modified the task in any way, perhaps bought an electric toothbrush or shaver for the sole reason to make the job easier? Have you changed the food you eat to reduce fine motor challenges? Changed the clothing you wear? Small changes can, when added up, result in a sizeable impact on your level of confidence, self-esteem, and independence.

Score each activity as indicated. For example, if your response is 'able to do alone', you would score one (1). If your response is 'unable to do at all', your score would be five (5). Add up your scores and note the grand total.

3. 6-Minute Walk Test

This is a straightforward test that measures how far you can walk in six minutes. How far you walk can give you a rough idea of your fitness level, how you compare to other people your age who don't have Parkinson's, and how much, if at all, your mobility is impaired.

For this test, you will need to mark out a 10-metre walkway that is relatively flat and unimpeded. Some people choose to use a long corridor, driveway, or sidewalk. You will also need a watch (or stopwatch) and good shoes. If you are uncertain about your balance, invite a buddy along to support and time you, but make sure there is no chatting - no distractions! Go as fast as you can for the full six minutes. If you are quite speedy and rack up a considerable number of laps, you may need to think of a way to record the number of laps accurately so you don't lose count.

Research shows that, on average, men in their early sixties without Parkinson's walk 572 metres while women in the same age group walk 538 metres. Men and women in their eighties walk 417 and 392 metres, respectively. These numbers will give you a rough idea of where you fall on this scale.

Again, it is good to know how you compare to others but, more importantly, how you compare to yourself when it comes time to re-test yourself.

4. Berg Balance Score

This is an assessment of your functional balance. It will give you a single score that can be standardised for comparison before and after your *10-Week Challenge*. This test may not be sensitive enough if your balance is very good. If you have concerns about your balance, however, it will give you a good indication of your risk of falls. There is extensive data on this test; however, it was not designed to be a self-assessment measure so bear that in mind when you compare your scores to the falls risk data. Despite that, I still think the self-assessment version is a good opportunity to gauge how you perform, especially to measure change over time if you are doing and scoring it the same way each time.

When you score yourself on this test, use the lowest achievable level. For example, if you can turn around in a full circle within six seconds, then you score yourself a 2 (able to turn 360 degrees safely, but slowly). When you have finished, add all the scores up and you will have a single score between zero and 56.

If you score between 41 and 56, you are considered to have a low falls risk. A score between 21 and 40 equals a medium falls risk and one 0 to 20 means that you have a high falls risk.

Getting started

What clothing and footwear should I wear when I do the exercises?
We encourage you to wear loose, comfortable clothing that breathes well. Layers may help if the ambient temperature varies or if you have difficulty regulating your body temperature. Your footwear needs to be supportive, such as trainers or walking shoes. No slippers or thongs!

What exercise equipment will I need?

There are a few inexpensive items that we recommend to make your *10-Week Challenge* more targeted, stimulating, and fun. If you have trouble getting all these items together yourself or prefer the convenience of having them pre-packaged and sent to you, visit http://www.pdwarrior.com/product and order on our secure online portal. We will send you a PD Warrior Home Starter Kit conveniently stocked with the following six items so you are ready to go.

What you need to get started:

- 2 lightweight scarves (silk, polyester, and tulle fabrics are best)
- Light resistance band (at least one metre long)
- Soft plush ball (20 cm diameter-plus)
- Adjustable height hurdle or foam block (20 cm long and 10 cm wide)
- Agility dots or non-slip floor markers (these provide visual markers for foot placement)
- Sturdy chair (preferably without arms)

To add an extra dimension to your program you can also add:

- Half-foam roller for thoracic extension (it also feels amazing!)
- Pedometer (to see how quickly you start clocking up the steps)
- Metronome (to improve your timing, perhaps even your dance moves!)
- Agility stones (these reduce the surface area you stand on to make some exercises more challenging - for advanced users only)
- Agility ladder (to provide a visual stepping target)
- Arm burner (for an upper limb and dual-tasking challenge as well as strength training effect)
- Artistic ribbons (colourful, fun, and to give you visual feedback about your arm movements)

Where should I do PD Warrior?

The beauty of PD Warrior is that, once you know the exercises and principles, you can do your home program virtually anywhere: in your living room, the local gym, even when travelling. To do PD Warrior safely and well, you must first consider how much room you will need. Most of the exercises require as much space as it takes for you to take a large step in every direction – forwards, sideways, and backwards – and not to have any furniture within a full arm span, plus a bit extra for good measure. Trust me, smacking your finger on a hard piece of furniture is neither fun nor effective for your program!

The next consideration is your flooring. Many of my clients clear out a space in the garage or use a spare bedroom or the lounge. These are all fine – just make sure there are no greasy marks or slippery mats, cords, or chair legs for you to slip on or trip over. PD Warrior uses powerful movements, not trips and spills, for maximum effect.

Make sure you have adequate space and ventilation. You want to be working hard and not be driven into another room because you are getting claustrophobic or overheating.

Finally, if you can access your favourite music during your workout, this will help to keep you motivated. A portable music player means there are no limitations to where you can work out. If you use an MP3 player, signing up for a music app can really leverage your access to good music. There are a huge number of excellent workout tracks to keep you inspired.

Remember, there is also the dual-tasking track that you can download if you are ready for Level 3 and need an extra challenge. Just go to the website to download the track: http://www.pdwarrior.com/how-to-get-started.

How often should I do the program?

Some of you will be employed full time, busy looking after grandkids, or perhaps involved in a large volume of leisure and sporting activities. That's great! We encourage you to **exercise every day** during the

10-Week Challenge. I was not kidding when I said the program was hard work and involves a serious commitment. If you are doing other exercise, like bike riding, bowls, or going to the gym, don't stop those activities. Add or modify the exercises to make them PD Warrior approved. Each time you do the PD Warrior circuit exercises or an exercise modified to PD Warrior standards, record your session in the back of this book.

The most important thing is to reflect on how hard you worked during the exercise. Tracking your perceived rate of exertion - RPE is really important so that you can start recognising how much effort your exercise and good movement should involve. When you have completed the *10-Week Challenge,* you can continue to do your PD Warrior exercises as often as you need to help you improve your regular sporting and leisure activities.

How hard should I be working?

You have read the section on high effort already, so you know what is expected of you. What you need to consider now are the logistics of doing a PD Warrior exercise. Each exercise is designed as a two-minute station. During the two-minute period, you should aim to work at 80 per cent effort. If you get tired, it's fine to take a break and resume the exercise. With all of the exercise stations, except for the warm-up and cool-down, you should be working towards a perceived exertion rate of 80 per cent maximum effort. This means that, when you move your arms and legs, you should be putting in 80 per cent effort to be powerful in your movements. That is big, energetic, and accurate in movement. It is better to do a few exercises in each circuit at 80 per cent effort than the whole two minutes at 50 per cent effort. If you are just starting out, walk your way through the exercises, building up to 80 per cent effort over the first few sessions. This will help you avoid injury and learn the exercise movements.

One strategy to help you with your effort level is to enlist a buddy to 'spot' you. Whether you are doing PD Warrior at home or in your local PD Warrior clinic, the job of your buddy is to give you feedback on how much effort you are putting into your exercise. Remember, the key to PD Warrior helping you with lasting change is to achieve high-effort movement. Your buddy can either do the exercises with you or watch and provide you with feedback as you start out. If you can do the full two minutes of the exercise when you first start, you are definitely not working at 80 per cent intensity.

If you are doing PD Warrior at home, it helps to have your buddy film you doing some or all of your exercises. There is nothing quite like watching yourself on video to reveal how much effort you're actually putting in. Because of the recalibration of normal movement commonly seen in Parkinson's, many people claim they feel ridiculous doing some of the exercises because they are designed to be powerful and performed on an exaggerated scale. Once I play their video though, they see what I see, which is often very different to what they feel the movement looked like. I find it is a really helpful demonstration tool. Try it out yourself. When was the last time you watched yourself walk?

Watching a video of yourself is not the same as watching yourself in the mirror. Using a mirror to give you feedback about your movements is not recommended. You want to see the best example of the exercise possible. If your movements are underpowered and underwhelming, you are just going to reinforce poor movement quality.

Keep focusing on the power involved in each exercise. Aim for symmetry, accuracy, and crisp, energetic movements. Each repetition counts. The exercises are not designed for you to get through them as quickly as possible. Think of the old saying: Quality before quantity.

For more information and advice on these concepts, review Chapter 4 and view the website, http://www.pdwarrior.com/how-to-get-started, for some examples of black belt PD Warriors showing some serious use of power!

What if one part of my body needs more attention?

If you have noticed more symptoms in one particular arm or leg, you may wish to focus on that limb more intensively during each exercise station. Make sure that this particular limb is leading the exercise in effort and scale. Focus on that limb and the rest of body will follow. The key concept is to remember that your movements need to be powerful and at 80 per cent effort.

You may also wish to double the repetitions on that side, especially if there is a marked difference from one side to the other.

What about my medication? Is there a better time to do the exercises?

Do you notice improvements in your mobility when you have taken your medication? If so, then I would recommend that you try and time doing your exercises when you are at your best, about 40 to 60 minutes after taking your medication.

If you have significant on/off periods, PD Warrior may help to improve your movements over time when you are off medication. It is not a good idea to do your exercises when you feel you are off. As well as being frustrating, it may also increase your risk of hurting yourself or falling over.

How can I modify the regular exercise I do to make it more effective?

If you are going to the gym, walking, running, or swimming regularly, there are ways to make these exercises more effective. Take walking: if you like to walk, that's great. What do you typically do? Go for a stroll around the block or power-walk up hills? While getting you on your feet and moving is important either way, here are three easy concepts you can add to any exercise to make it more effective and help your brain fitness.

Using the walking example, adding exaggerated power movements to the quality of your walking, both arm swing and stride length, can improve the amplitude of all of your movements. By increasing the intensity of your walking and making it energetic and vigorous, even if you only put the effort in between every second light post, the sprint training will help with general fitness as well as brain fitness.

In fact, short interval-based training programs have been shown to have many benefits over longer, more consistently paced exercise.

Finally, consider the complexity of the walking. Safety is obviously something you need to consider to prevent falls and injury, but consider increasing the complexity of your walking by adding a dual task while you are performing your high-effort intervals. This can be another motor task, like moving coins back and forth from one pocket to the other, or a mental task like spelling your full name backwards. Simply by making your usual walking more complex, you are challenging your brain a little bit more and making it react to the stimulation.

If you cycle, these same concepts apply. Aim for a baseline revolutions per minute (RPM) of 80 and introduce some sprints. See if you can exceed 100 RPM. If you can, then add a mental challenge - all the while keeping your RPM over 80. Adding this additional complexity will make a huge difference to your regular exercise program.

There are a few activities that might need a little more creativity in order to adapt - Pilates and yoga are two such examples. These types of exercise have been developed for other reasons, but you can still add elements of power, amplitude, and complexity when you are doing the exercises.

Recreational dancing and dancing classes for Parkinson's are also a great way to stay in shape and keep moving. Elements of PD Warrior can be introduced to the choreography, and there will be an element of complexity to the dance moves.

Just remember that there is a difference between training for neuroplastic change and general exercise principles. If you are training for positive neuroplastic change, then you need all the elements of PD Warrior in your exercise program. If you are training for general exercise or recreation and enjoy what you are doing, then keep doing it!

If you are training for positive neuroplastic change, then you need all the elements of PD Warrior in your exercise program.

7

Common Misperceptions

Before PD Warrior became an international program, people would call up saying they were coming to Sydney and wanted to book an intensive PD Warrior program. It delighted me to know that PD Warrior had achieved such widespread exposure, especially coming from people living in the most remote locations; however, it was important to explain that PD Warrior isn't guaranteed to work for everyone. Over time, I identified half a dozen common misperceptions that people have about the PD Warrior program.

Six common misperceptions people have regarding PD Warrior

1. PD Warrior will work for me because it helps everyone with Parkinson's.
2. My symptoms aren't severe enough for PD Warrior to have any real benefit.
3. The exercises are so easy that I can afford to push myself a lot harder than I'm being asked to.

4. I've made progress so I can skip a few workouts.
5. I'm already doing an exercise program and one exercise is as good as another.
6. I don't need to track my progress every time; I have a pretty good idea how I'm doing.

Let's take a closer look at each of these.

1. **PD Warrior will work for me because it helps everyone with Parkinson's.**

First of all, PD Warrior is designed for people who have idiopathic and early stage Parkinson's. If your symptoms are atypical and you haven't responded well to medication, then PD Warrior may not help you as much. If you are fairly advanced, PD Warrior may not be the best program for you and certainly not when done in isolation without a PD Warrior Instructor supporting you. You need to be assessed as eligible for PD Warrior in order to attend one of the circuit classes. If you have chosen to do a DIY program through this book, clearly we can't assess your eligibility.

PD Warrior is designed for people who already have a reasonable level of fitness or some basic fitness routine. PD Warrior is quite a vigorous exercise approach and is not for the faint-hearted. If you don't exercise at all, it doesn't mean that PD Warrior is not appropriate for you. You just need to be careful, as you would need to be when starting any new exercise program.

In order to get the most out of the PD Warrior program, it's critical to first learn its underlying principles. Most of our clients start by coming into a PD Warrior centre at least two or three times for individual sessions in order to learn and fully appreciate the principles, how to move and how to progress. This book can only tell you how to do the exercises. It is the feedback you get from your instructor (and a really good buddy) that makes the difference between an average program and a successful one.

A buddy is very important in providing you with feedback, but they need to know what to focus their feedback on, not just how to give it. This is why PD Warrior is best delivered by health professionals who have been specially trained as instructors. Each instructor knows how to tailor the program to you by teasing out the most effective movement strategies for you for maximum effect. They will also be able to provide you with tips to improve your technique, help to clarify some of the exercises, and show you ways to avoid injuring yourself.

PD Warrior can involve multidimensional movements designed to test your effort levels, balance, flexibility, strength, fitness, and coordination. They can also help to train your buddy to work effectively with you.

It is important when choosing to proceed with the DIY program that you be sensible and use your best judgement as to whether you think PD Warrior is suitable for you.

2. **My symptoms aren't severe enough for PD Warrior to have any real benefit.**

Even if you have just been diagnosed, chances are you have had symptoms, even sub-clinical ones, for several years before being diagnosed and that you are not doing all the things you could be. Convincing someone to start PD Warrior is not difficult once they have been assessed, as the assessment process makes those areas needing improvement very apparent. Convincing someone that they need to work harder when they don't feel the need is quite a different story. I have not met a PD Warrior yet who has not impressed themselves when they really apply the PD Warrior principles. PD Warrior is not rocket science, but you do need to adhere to the seven core principles to get the most out of the program. One of the principles is that you need to work hard - harder than you have in a long time.

Most people I meet think that because they exercise regularly, they already know how to work hard at it. I think you would be amazed at how hard you can really work, and when you start working hard, how well you start to move. Even the extremely fit people I meet are stunned to discover how small and slow their movements actually are when they begin the PD Warrior exercises. Do not be fooled into thinking that because you are relatively fit, newly diagnosed, or still considered 'mild', PD Warrior is going to be easy. If you find doing PD Warrior is easy, then you are not doing it right!

It should always be hard enough that you can JUST do the exercise. Remember the Goldilocks Concept. The minute you master a level, you must advance yourself to the next level. You cannot afford to get comfortable at any level and coast, because at that point your brain stops learning and you are wasting potential opportunities.

3. **The exercises are so easy that I can afford to push myself a lot harder than I'm being asked to.**

Some people mistakenly assume PD Warrior is easy and so they overdo it and hurt themselves. This is one reason why I like to train people individually for a few sessions before letting them loose in a PD Warrior circuit. PD Warrior, when done well, involves strong, powerful, full-body movements. It also encourages you to use the full range of motion in your arms and legs. If you have not moved in that range for a long time, you need to be careful adding any power to your movements to avoid injury.

Every PD Warrior needs to ease into the program at first. Yes, we ask you to work hard; yes, we ask you to be powerful; but always safely, to your limits, and never to the point of injury. If you are doing this program at home for the first time, please be careful during your first few sessions to make sure you don't risk injuring yourself. We are not there to correct your movements and improve your technique, so if anything niggles, stop doing the exercise and read the instructions again.

4. **I've made progress so I can skip a few workouts.**

We call this falling off the wagon. It doesn't usually happen during the *10-Week Challenge* but more often after that phase of the program has finished and colleagues, family, and friends have begun commenting on the great results you've achieved. It is easy to get complacent at this stage. Falling off the wagon can happen for many reasons, the most common being that the benefits of the program are not fully understood, or a better offer comes up, such as going away on holidays.

Parkinson's doesn't go on holidays;
exercise needs to be for life.

PD Warrior is not a quick fix or a cure – it is a lifestyle choice. What PD Warrior offers you is a way to take charge of your Parkinson's and slow down the progression of your symptoms. Parkinson's does not take a holiday and so neither can you. If you want to move the best you can move, feel the best you can feel, and live the best life you can live every single day, you must work at it every single day. Fighting the symptoms of Parkinson's through exercise, especially through the PD Warrior program, is a commitment for life, well beyond the first *10-Week Challenge.*

PD Warrior is an exercise behaviour strategy. Improving with PD Warrior is arguably the easy part – it is much harder to stick to it. Please keep that in mind when you set your goals.

REPEAT: I AM A PD WARRIOR FOR LIFE!

Being a PD Warrior for life doesn't mean adopting a regimented program that is going to wear you into the ground. The idea is to use the *10-Week Challenge* as an opportunity to commit to yourself: committing to change bad habits, committing to forgive yourself if you slip up, and committing to asking for help when you are struggling to keep on track. The *10-Week Challenge* has created some inspiring stories. Now it's time to write your own!

5. **I'm already doing an exercise program and one exercise is as good as another.**

If you already have a regular exercise program, congratulations! You are already on your way to fighting the symptoms of Parkinson's. PD Warrior can refine some of your current exercises to target the symptoms of Parkinson's more specifically and help you see results more efficiently in the areas you need to work on.

Exercise programs such as Pilates and yoga definitely have their place in Parkinson's treatment, especially in terms of improving strength and flexibility, which can become secondary problems. However, they do not work you hard enough in terms of driving your motor output. Loss of motor output in Parkinson's is one of the primary problems leading to slow and small movements. If you enjoy doing Pilates and yoga, certainly continue, but if the major symptoms of your Parkinson's are movements that are slow and small or tremor dominant, I would recommend that you start focusing more on exercise methods that promote greater motor output.

If you go to the gym regularly for strength and resistance training, great! This, too, has a place in the treatment of your Parkinson's and for many other reasons, including your general health, bone health, metabolic health, and maintaining a healthy weight range. There is some evidence to suggest that strength and resistance exercises can improve the small movements discussed above, however, for the same reasons mentioned before, strength and resistance training alone will not give you the best results.

People also come in who have a passion for jogging, walking, cycling, and swimming. I love these as baseline exercises because they can all be easily modified to target Parkinson's more specifically. Repetitive tasks such as cycling and swimming rarely improve skill acquisition and motor learning, especially if you have been doing them for a long time. You likely find the movements easy to do and, when you exercise, you do it at your own pace. This does not promote increased motor output or skill acquisition because you have become too accomplished at the task. If you have found that you are starting to have more difficulty with such repetitive tasks as swimming and cycling, perhaps falling behind your buddies or feeling that it's begun to take more effort than before, PD Warrior may be able to help.

By mixing up your program, PD Warrior shakes your body off the path leading to smaller and slower movements. PD Warrior is a platform that enables you to learn challenging, novel, and intense exercises that reflect functional activities you typically do during the day. All of our exercises are designed to override smaller, slower movements by generating effort and increased motor output. By all means keep cycling, jogging, and swimming. Our goal is to get you to work a bit harder and more powerfully.

PD Warrior is a platform that enables you to learn challenging, novel, and intense exercises that reflect functional activities you typically do during the day.

---

6. **I don't need to track my progress every time; I have a pretty good idea how I'm doing.**

It is so important to document your sessions and the effort level you use. If you don't record it, you can't track it. If you can't track it, then you can't see how you are improving. This is especially important if your symptoms are very mild and you are not yet convinced that this program is really for you. Keeping a record of your exercise will demonstrate in black and white what you have accomplished and how you are progressing through the program. It will also make the effect glaringly obvious when you miss a day or two, and may help to keep you on track to reaching your goals.

Recording your exercise sessions should also help you plan your diary and keep exercise as a high priority, so make sure you keep your exercise record up to date. There are *10-Week Challenge* record sheets available in the back of this book. You can also get them from the website by registering at http://www.pdwarrior.com/10-week-challenge, when you sign up for the weekly support emails.

8

How to Stay Motivated

'Obstacles are those frightful things you see
when you take your eyes off your goal.' **Henry Ford**

The benefits of regular exercise have been well documented, both for your general health and specifically for Parkinson's. We all know that we should probably exercise more, and if you find exercise challenging, this section is possibly more relevant for you. Perhaps there has never been an exercise that you enjoyed, or one that you could happily stick to. Starting and sticking with an exercise program is not always easy, especially if exercise is a foreign concept, however, there are a few strategies that you can put in place early to make sure that you give the *10-Week Challenge* a really good go. Any habit can be broken in three weeks, so just imagine what you can do in ten!

Be realistic and prepare for obstacles

Expect some stumbles and setbacks and start thinking about how to renew your energy and get back on track when they happen. Answer these questions, and rate your answer on a scale from 0 to 10:

1. How confident are you that you will stick to the *10-Week Challenge*? (10 being extremely confident and 0 being not confident at all)
2. How do you rate the importance of exercise right now? (10 being extremely important and 0 being not important at all)

With each of your scores, have a think about what might be stopping you from rating higher. What would have to happen for your score to increase?

Being prepared and knowing the pitfalls and challenges ahead before you start can help you to prepare strategies to be successful.

If-Then Technique

A good technique to consider at this point is the if-then technique: *'If* x happens, *then* I will do y. Declare what has to happen in order for you to exercise, as well as where, when, and with whom, and you are likely to be much more successful. There is a large body of literature exploring the relationship between intending to exercise and actually exercising. Many individuals fail to link intent to behaviour.

> *If I am too tired to exercise, then I will review my reasons to exercise for some inspiration.*

> *If I don't feel like exercising, then I will call my buddy to help motivate me.*

A more positive way to frame these statements might be:

> *If it is 6 am, then I will do 20 minutes of PD Warrior.*

Also reframing a statement like 'I will work out more' into something specific, such as 'I will go for a power march for 40 minutes in the park on Mondays, Wednesdays, and Fridays after work', suggests that you are two to three times more likely to follow through and succeed than if you don't use an if-then plan.

Make exercise a regular part of your day

What does that actually mean? It means that you need to build it into your day so that it is not left to the last minute or discarded because you get a better offer. Schedule your exercise into your day so that it has top priority. This is your health we are talking about and no one else can do your exercise for you. Medication can only do so much.

Learn to prioritise your exercise and say no to distractions. The *10-Week Challenge* is best done without bisecting it with a holiday or major disruption. Choose a start date that is going to give you the best chance of completing the 10 weeks uninterrupted, but don't let that become a reason for procrastinating. Your life and wellbeing are more important, aren't they? Make sure that you establish an exercise routine and be disciplined.

If you are really busy, you might find breaking your program down into several manageable 10-minute chunks suits you better. There is good evidence to show that this is still effective to receive a cardiovascular and strength training. I think it is fine for training motor output and re-wiring your brain too. Perhaps you might schedule a few exercises for when you wake up in the morning, another round at mid-morning, lunch, mid-afternoon, and then evening. See what works best for you with your lifestyle and medication schedule, but make sure you plan it and record it.

If you are particularly short of time, avoid the temptation to throw in the towel completely. Do what you have time to do. Something is better than nothing at all. Even five minutes of PD Warrior exercises done well may yield results when done consistently, if not as much as employing the entire program as recommended.

If you continually find yourself short of time, ask yourself honestly whether you have truly put your exercise program at the top of your priority list. Is everything else you're doing *really* as important to your wellbeing?

Goal Setting

Planning your goals well, believing in yourself, and being able to reflect on your progress may all sound like fairly abstract concepts, but they are crucial to help you to achieve your best results, not just from the *10-Week Challenge*, but also from longer-term exercise activities.

Planning your goals is essential. If you don't have a specific goal to guide you to the end of your journey, it's like not having a road map. You could end up anywhere or nowhere at all. You will be directionless. Think about where you want to go. Spend a bit of time reflecting on why you have perhaps not achieved goals in the past. Were they too vague? Did they not establish a certain timeframe? Goals, to be effective, must have structure. Identifying any common obstacles now can stop you getting derailed.

As well as providing a structure, setting worthwhile and salient goals can be incredibly exciting. Goals boost self-confidence when achieved, especially when short-term achievements are linked to longer-term goals and the 'big picture'. Goal setting is not just an art. There is also a little science to it.

Are you familiar with the SMART mnemonic? Successful people use this as a way to set goals and stay focused. While it may vary slightly, SMART essentially stands for the same thing:

S	=	**Specific**
M	=	**Measurable**
A	=	**Attainable**
R	=	**Realistic**
T	=	**Timely**

Start by listing the What, Why, and How of your goal:

Specific: *I want to roll in bed without help.*
  If you can't measure it, you can't manage it. Choose a goal with measurable progress and concrete criteria:

Measurable: *I want to walk one kilometre in 15 minutes.*
Make sure your goal will challenge you but is not so far out of your reach that you won't commit to seeing it through.

Attainable: *I want to be comfortable signing my own name in public.*
Set the bar high enough for its achievement to feel satisfying. Too difficult sets the stage for failure, but too low sends the message that you aren't very capable.

Realistic: *I want to order steak when we go out to dinner and not feel self-conscious cutting it up.*
A specific timeframe makes you feel more accountable. The timeframe must be measurable, attainable, and realistic.

Timely: *I want to return to playing 18 holes of golf in 10 weeks.*
The 10-Week Challenge is a terrific (and realistic) timeframe for your shorter-term goals.

Goal setting is more fun and also more effective if you establish rewards for your achievements. When you reach a goal that you've set for yourself, it is important to recognise the implications of having reached it - *and celebrate!* Each small win makes your brain do a little happy dance and that happy dance represents a little drop of dopamine. Rewards can be simple, like taking yourself shopping or to the movies - whatever is your cup of tea.

Rewarding yourself is even better when you let others reward you too. Seek support from loved ones as well as the PD Warrior Community on the PD Warrior Facebook page. The page is where other PD Warriors record their wins, both big and small, and their moments of brilliance, insight, and inspiration. Help inspire others by letting them celebrate your successes on our Facebook page.

One thing to remember when setting goals is that, in the early stages of Parkinson's, you are likely to see reversal of some of your symptoms and sometimes substantial improvements. It can be very exciting. But it is important to understand that Parkinson's is a progressive condition and no treatment, including PD Warrior, can change that. Your window of symptom reversibility starts to lessen as your condition progresses.

Don't let that discourage you. PD Warrior, at its best, can reverse some of your symptoms and definitely help you to move better in the early stages. At the very least, it will make you fitter, stronger, and more confident in yourself as well, all while it helps to slow your symptom progression down. Because of the progressive nature of Parkinson's, maintaining your current functional capacity and ability over a set period of time is to be considered a victory, something to be celebrated! Don't let anyone scoff at or undermine these achievements.

Setting your goals

OK, are you ready? Have you registered for the *10-Week Challenge* on the website? If you haven't registered already, sign up now so that you have everything you need. Sign up here: www.pdwarrior. com/10-week-challenge. You will also find a copy of this information in the back of the book, from page 155.

It might also be helpful to take a few moments to review the PDQ-8 and SPDDS self-assessment sheets that you completed. They will help to identify challenges you currently face and goals that you may wish to work towards.

This next step requires some thoughtful consideration. It's time to determine a single long-term goal and three shorter-term goals to help you to achieve this.

Your **long-term goal** is your 'big picture' goal. Examples of this might be Pat who wanted to get back to playing tennis, or Cindy who wanted to tick off a trip to Antarctica that was on her bucket list. Both of these ladies achieved their goals but they took many months to achieve. You might achieve your long-term goal during the *10-Week Challenge* but it usually takes more time. It might also be an ongoing goal. Peter wanted to stay fit enough to keep up with his mates when they went cycling and Bob wanted to stay at work for another twelve months.

Think about your current lifestyle. Are there any tasks or activities that you've either modified or stopped doing altogether that you'd love to see yourself achieve again? What is your long-term goal? Write it down on your goal sheet on page 174.

Your **short-term goals** are components of your long-term goal. For Pat, in order to get back to tennis, she needed to improve her service motion. Her short-term goals were built around regaining full, pain-free range of movement at the shoulder, a strong grip to hold the tennis racquet, and knowing what moving at 80 per cent of her RPE felt like. For Cindy, one of her short-term goals was to be fit enough to walk over 500 metres in ten minutes while wearing heavy snow boots. These short-term goals were designed to help these two women achieve their 'big picture' goal and were achievable during the *10-Week Challenge.*

What are your top three **short-term** goals?

When you are happy with your goals, write them on your goal sheet. I would also recommend that you post your goals somewhere obvious where you will see them every day, like next to the bathroom mirror.

Next, write down the reasons why you have chosen to do PD Warrior and why you believe this program will help you to achieve your goals.

What are your beliefs around exercise? I want you to take a moment now to reflect on what exercise means to you. If it is something you love doing and have always done, then you have already developed strong exercise behaviour patterns. If you are new to exercise, sceptical, or even rebellious at some sub-conscious level, it is a step forward to recognise this now, to identify the challenges you face. Identifying them is the first step to overcoming them.

If you can link doing exercise to achieving what is precious to you, it will make it that much easier to fire up your motivation when you need a bit of a boost. Taking a few moments to complete your reasons to exercise will help you do this. Write down your thoughts on general exercise and how it and PD Warrior are going to help you achieve your goals. Keep this handy and review it anytime you feel your motivation needs a shot in the arm.

To believe in PD Warrior is to believe in yourself. PD Warrior is the vehicle, the catalyst, to motivate and assist you to make those positive changes and achieve your goals. 'You can lead a horse to water, but you can't make it drink.' PD Warrior is the water and this book is leading you to it, but you have to actually want to drink the water – to make the change – and that means you have to want to do the exercises in order to reap the benefits and stay ahead of the progression of your symptoms as much as you can. A huge achievement takes a huge commitment. And it can bring huge rewards.

To get the most out of your program, you must believe that PD Warrior will help you make those changes. The journey is going to be challenging. It is challenging for every successful PD Warrior. If you are not yet convinced that general exercise and the PD Warrior program are going to help you get your life back by the time you finish reading this book, find a PD Warrior Instructor and go and see them.

You can do it. And PD Warrior is here to help you, to see you through.

Get a buddy

We all need support in life. Enlisting a buddy is like having your very own motivational coach, and is a tried and tested method to help you stick to your program. They are there as much to make your exercise sessions more stimulating, more fun, and more enjoyable as to provide you with objective feedback about your ongoing progress. Often, a buddy gets just as much out of the shared experience as their partner. Your buddy will also keep you on track when you are having 'one of those days' – and they do happen. They happen to all of us. If you have scheduled exercise sessions with a buddy who is enthusiastic and vested in your success, it can mean the difference between staying the course and dropping out. You are far more likely to stick to it when cancelling a session means cancelling with them, after they've scheduled time to spend working with you.

Having a buddy can also provide a competitive edge to your sessions and help you to work that little bit harder. Your buddy needn't be a passive observer just watching you exercise. They can participate with you, and get a good workout, regardless of whether they have Parkinson's or not.

How do you pick your buddy? It helps to pick someone convenient, like your spouse, a son or daughter, or a friend. Whoever you choose, make sure that they know up front that you are asking them to make a serious commitment to helping you. That means time and energy. This is a really good reason to schedule your exercise sessions so that they're convenient to you both.

Your buddy is most important in the early stages when you may not know your potential, how hard you can work, how powerful your movements can be, or how much you can upscale the size of your movements. I typically recommend training with your buddy every day in the first week. Over time, you probably won't need as much help from them and might only need to work out with them every couple of days. (You'll still need to work out every day, remember!)

Your buddy is most important in the early stages when you may not know your potential.

The role of your buddy is to provide you with constructive feedback, even when you don't want to hear it. Constructive feedback is designed to improve the way you do your exercises, not tear you to shreds. For this reason, it is important to choose someone supportive, someone that you trust, so that you trust the feedback they are giving you. It is always a good idea to lay some ground rules in the early stages to make sure that training with your buddy is an uplifting experience, not one that shakes your confidence.

Rules for your buddy (Have them read this section.)

Dear Buddy,

You have agreed to support _____ in their *10-Week Challenge*. Your role is to assist your buddy to reach their PD Warrior potential by providing feedback, motivation, and encouragement throughout the full 10 weeks of the program. Please review the goals your buddy has set so that you can help your buddy to achieve these during the program. Schedule mutually convenient exercise sessions in advance and stick to them. Sessions can include PD Warrior exercises as well as general exercise and activities. You are, of course, invited to join your buddy in working out during these sessions.

Here is some advice on providing feedback to your buddy:

1. If you can't think of a constructive purpose for giving feedback, don't give any.
2. Focus on being objective and encouraging rather than judgemental, and maintain dignity and respect in your comments.
3. Be aware of feedback overload. Providing too much feedback can be counter-productive.
4. Be very concise and specific about the feedback and any suggestions you give.
5. Keep personal feelings under control. Feelings of anger or frustration will be evident in your tone.
6. Focus on your buddy's behaviour and the quality of their exercise, not them as a person.
7. Be direct; don't beat around the bush.
8. Agree on targets and outcomes before the session starts.

Rules for you
1. Be open to feedback and ask for it regularly.
2. Try to take the feedback on board and improve your actions because of it.
3. Accept the possibility that someone else can see things in your exercise performance that you can't.
4. Try not to be defensive.
5. Ask for a demonstration or clarification if you do not understand.

Music

I cannot say enough about music and how having the right kind of music can mean the difference between enjoying a session and enduring it. There's a reason why music with a strong beat and rhythm is played in just about every gym in the world. Music not only gets you moving to a beat, keeping you from slowing down, but it also lifts your spirits and keeps you motivated, long after you might otherwise have pulled the pin.

Music is a huge part of all our PD Warrior sessions and I strongly encourage you to get your favourite songs ready. At the risk of having you mock my music choices, I have listed some of my favourite songs to accompany PD Warrior exercises. These have catchy tunes and a beat range that falls between 100 to 150 beats per minute, which is a good brisk pace. Alternatively, make up your own favourite playlist or get out your favourite CD. Do whatever you need to get started!

My favourite playlist:

SONG	ARTIST
Staying Alive	Bee Gees
Black Betty	Ram Jam
Another One Bites the Dust	Queen
I Will Survive	Gloria Gaynor
Beat It	Michael Jackson
Eye of the Tiger	Survivor
Rebel Yell	Billy Idol
Thunderstruck	AC/DC
Paint It Black	The Rolling Stones
Born to Be Wild	Steppenwolf
Hurricane	Bob Dylan
The Rockafeller Skank	Fatboy Slim
Boom Boom Pow	Black Eyed Peas
Laura	Scissor Sisters
Maneater	Nelly Furtado
Hit the Road, Jack	Ray Charles
Suicide Blonde	INXS
Bamboleo	Gypsy Kings
Long Train Running	The Doobie Brothers
Drive My Car	The Beatles
Hot Stuff	Donna Summer

Start recording and tracking in your diary

There are few things more motivating than watching your workout log increase in line with your results. That's why you'll find a *10-Week Challenge* diary in the back of the book. You will also have a copy emailed to you when you register for the *10-Week Challenge*. Record each of your sessions in the diary, even if it's only a 10-minute session. You want to be able to add up the total number of minutes you've spent exercising at the end of every week.

During the *10-Week Challenge,* your aim is to complete at least 60 minutes of good quality exercise each day. This is not limited solely to PD Warrior exercises – it may also include your daily walk, session at the gym, gardening, whatever. What is important though is that, if you are not doing PD Warrior exercises specifically, you are thinking about how to integrate the principles of PD Warrior into any other exercise that you do.

If you are going for a walk, go for a PD Warrior power march. If you are working out at the gym, use the bike or treadmill for interval sprints and work on your speed, rather than resistance. If you are gardening, be as Warrior-like as you can be in all your movements. (Those weeds won't stand a chance!)

Be powerful. You are now a PD Warrior in all that you do.

Remember: each minute, each repetition, each exercise counts. If you only have five minutes to work out, make them five strenuous minutes, not simply five minutes spent trying to get your exercises done as quickly as possible.

I'm still struggling. What else can I do?

So far you've set your goals, enlisted a buddy, scheduled your exercise, cleared a space, and got your music playlist organised. And, yet, your motivation is waning. Don't worry! This is perfectly normal. PD Warrior is a hard slog and can make vegging on the couch seem very appealing.

If you find yourself in a hole, the first thing to do is stop diggin'.
– Old farmer's advice

If you have been going at it for a while, take a break. Take a day or two to have a rest and re-energise before getting back into it. Try not to leave it more than two days though as it will become harder to motivate yourself. While you're taking a break, review your progress log. That will give you a sharper, clearer idea of what you really have accomplished so far and make you eager to continue.

Change your perspective. Movement is an amazing privilege that we able-bodied individuals often take for granted. *Able-bodied?* Well, you may consider your movements to be poor, but there is always someone out there who cannot move as well as you can. Believe me, I know. As a neurological physiotherapist, I am reminded every day to be thankful for the movement I have and not to waste a precious moment. What those others wouldn't do to be able to move like you!

Movement is an amazing privilege. Consider the movement ability that you have as a blessing. Fight hard to keep it as long as you can.

Consider the movement ability that you have as a blessing. Fight - *fight hard* - to keep it as long as you can and don't give up because it is hard work. PD Warrior can be a tough journey, but I can assure you that not doing PD Warrior will likely be harder in the long term.

Finally, mix it up a bit. We all love a bit of variety and fun. Have you got grandkids who will do the exercises with you to music, maybe The Wiggles? What about a mate who will go to the park with you? Get a local group together and have a little friendly PD Warrior competition. Fun is crucial to keeping you going. What are you waiting for? Get creative!

9

The 10–Week Challenge

'Good enough never is.'

Debbi Fields

The *10-Week Challenge* was developed to help structure your program so that you can get the best out of PD Warrior. As well as delivering the education that you need to continue with the program, the PD Warrior *10-Week Challenge* promotes good exercise behaviours that will sustain you after you finish.

I would again encourage you to register for the *10-Week Challenge* on our website. Visit http://www.pdwarrior.com/10-week-challenge and enter your email address. In addition to the PD Warrior exercises, there are focus points for you to consider each week. These are really important to help you stay on track as well as assist you in creating good exercise behaviours for long-term change. I suggest you work your way through each week and if you encounter any problems, don't hesitate to get in touch with your PD Warrior Instructor, or hop on the Facebook page.

You are ready to get started if:

1. You've been cleared by a PD Warrior Instructor or health professional to start the program.
2. You've completed the self-assessment section and recorded your results.
3. You've identified your goals for the program, both short and long term.
4. You have acknowledged your reasons for doing PD Warrior on the goal page.
5. You're unaware of any injuries or health reasons that might prevent you from exercising.
6. You've sourced all the equipment you need and cleared out a space.
7. You've registered your *10-Week Challenge* by posting on the Facebook page.

If you've done all the above, let's get started!

WEEK 1

Welcome to the PD Warrior exercise program.

I want you to record your daily activities by starting an activity diary. For suggestions on what you need to record, refer to the activity log at the back of this book on page 173.

How much activity are you doing at the moment? Activity is anything that involves use of energy or incidental exercise: gardening, walking, shopping, housework, outings, etc. What about regular exercise? Record all of your exercise, and the level of effort you put into your exercise each time. Pop it all down in your diary. Some people find using a pedometer or activity tracker to be a good way to measure their steps from when they rise in the morning until when they go to bed at night. A great goal is 10,000 steps per day. How many steps do you average now?

What you want to get from your first week is a rough idea of how much activity you average each day. At the end of the first week, record your feelings about exercise and your efforts.

I feel:

E.g., I feel excited about the PD Warrior journey ahead of me.

_____

_____

_____

_____

I achieved:

E.g., I managed to start working at 80% effort by the
end of the week.

_____

_____

_____

_____

I am most proud of:

E.g., This week I completed my program every single day.

_____

_____

_____

_____

I averaged about _____ minutes of activity / steps each
day this week.

WEEK 2

If you have not already done so, now is a good time to solicit some reaction from your buddy. Your buddy will be able to give you feedback on your exercises as well as how you are doing in other general activities, perhaps even on your mood. Make sure your buddy understands that you are asking for *constructive* feedback!

You're not limited to one buddy. Buddies can come from many areas and they do not only have to be physical buddies. If you enlist on our Facebook page, you can sign up with heaps of other people who are also doing their PD Warrior *10-Week Challenge*. You are never alone when you are a PD Warrior!

To meet a buddy or make a comment, visit the PD Warrior Facebook page at http://www.facebook.com/PDWarriorProgram. Make sure to 'like' the page so that you can keep up to date with the latest helpful hints and new stories.

At the end of the second week, record your feelings about your buddy, your exercise, and your efforts.

My buddy is:

_____

_____

_____

_____

My buddy helps me most with:

_____

_____

_____

_____

The best part about doing the PD Warrior exercises is:

_____

_____

_____

_____

WEEK 3

By Week 3, you should be starting to feel comfortable with the exercises in the PD Warrior program, especially your homework. This week is a good opportunity to start working on your overall effort level during the exercise. Use the PD Warrior RPE scale on page 40 to help you work out where you sit on the effort scale. Are you achieving 80% effort yet? Make sure to record this in the back of the book.

If you are having trouble with any of the exercises or need more of a visual clarification, talk to your PD Warrior Instructor or visit the PD Warrior website, http://www.pdwarrior.com, where the exercises are available to view by video in the *Get Started* section.

At the end of the third week, record your feelings about exercise and your efforts.

When I am working at 80% effort, I feel like:

_____

_____

_____

_____

My main reason to exercise is:

_____

_____

_____

_____

My favourite PD Warrior exercise is ... because ...

_____

_____

_____

_____

WEEK 4

Have you had any 'Wow!' moments yet? Usually by this stage, if you have been doing PD Warrior consistently and at the right effort level, you will start to experience improvement in some of your movements. Make sure to write these 'Wow!' moments here and please post them on the Facebook page to help inspire others.

If you don't feel like you are making enough progress, check out your record sheet to determine how much effort you're putting into the program. If you're working hard, don't worry. Keep working at it and the results should come.

Remember, your 'Wow!' moments can be little things, like managing to do your buttons up in half the time, right through to the big things, like going for a bushwalk for the first time in two years. When you have a 'Wow!' moment, no matter how small, shout it out and celebrate! Share the elation! It's like fertiliser – it can't do any good if you keep it locked away.

At the end of the fourth week, record your feelings about exercise and your efforts.

My first 'Wow!' moment was:

_____

_____

_____

_____

The most inspiring aspect of PD Warrior is:

_____

_____

_____

_____

I am confident that PD Warrior is going to help me achieve the following:

_____

_____

_____

_____

WEEK 5

Congratulations! You are halfway through the *10-Week Challenge* now!

Start thinking more and more about how to apply the principles of PD Warrior to your everyday activities. You should be moving with purpose and power in all of these activities. I want you to feel like you are standing taller, standing prouder – standing like a warrior fighting Parkinson's.

Introduce Power and as much full movement / High Effort as you can into all your daily activities. This includes opening doors, walking up the stairs, emptying the dishwasher, even turning the pages of the newspaper. (Not too much power on that last one!) Focus on generating Power and High Effort in all your movements.

At the end of the fifth week, record your feelings about exercise and your efforts.

This week I worked on Power and High Effort when doing the following activities:

_____

_____

_____

_____

This week I surprised myself by achieving:

_____

_____

_____

_____

When I am struggling to get motivated, I find that doing this helps me:

_____

_____

_____

_____

WEEK 6

If you have stopped keeping your activity diary, dig it out now.

Record all of your daily activities on at least three days this week in your activity diary. How much activity are you doing now? Are you doing more regular exercise? If you are doing PD Warrior regularly, you should be achieving at least 60 minutes of exercise on most days of the week. If you started using a pedometer, jot down the number of steps you're taking this week. If you have invested in an activity tracker, you might find this gives you more accurate results and more motivation.

How much exercise did you do each day this week and how does it compare to the first week of the challenge?

You should notice a dramatic increase in your overall activity levels. If you were suffering with fatigue, this should be improving and you should be feeling more powerful and more warrior-like in your everyday movements.

At the end of the sixth week, record your feelings about exercise and your efforts.

I am feeling better about dealing with my Parkinson's because:

_____

_____

_____

_____

I am doing **60** minutes of exercise on _____ days of the week.

My level of fatigue is: same / better / worse.

I have started doing these activities again:

_____

_____

_____

_____

I averaged about _____ minutes of activity/ steps each day this week.

WEEK 7

Remember back to the goals that you wrote at the beginning of the 10 Week Challenge. How are you going? Now is a good time to reflect on whether your goals are right for you or do they need some adjusting. Were the goal that your wrote down realistic? Have you measured up against them and do they need to be tweaked, perhaps made harder? How many of them are you likely to achieve in the *10 Week Challenge*?

What about your long-term goals? 10 weeks is enough to get you into peak physical condition. but what goals do you want to achieve in the longer term? What does the big picture look like to you?

I am hoping that by now, you are seeing a bigger future and bigger picture... don't be afraid to write this down!

Parkinson's is only part of you, don't let it define you.

Don't forget, we would love to hear from you.

Are you on track with your goals or do you need a bit of help? Please tell us how you are going on the Facebook page.

At the end of this seventh week, how much have you learnt about the principles of PD Warrior?

The four pillars of PD Warrior are:

1. _____
2. _____
3. _____
4. _____

Why is life–long exercise so important for managing Parkinson's?

_____

_____

_____

_____

What are the seven core principles of PD Warrior and why are they important?

1. _____
2. _____
3. _____
4. _____
5. _____
6. _____
7. _____

This is the goal I am most likely to achieve or have achieved already in the 10 Week Challenge:

_____

_____

_____

WEEK 8

This is a good opportunity, as you come towards the pointy end of the program, to review what you have learnt so far doing PD Warrior.

1. What is the most important lesson you have learnt so far in PD Warrior?

_____

_____

_____

2. Has your overall activity level improved? Are you thinking about ways to keep it up after the PD Warrior *10-Week Challenge*? If so, how?

_____

_____

_____

3. What activities have you started integrating PD Warrior principles into regularly?

_____

_____

_____

4. Are you feeling motivated and in control of your Parkinson's?

_____

_____

_____

5. **Exercise is medicine and is best taken as a daily dose.** Are you starting to feel the benefits of your increased commitment to yourself, your health, and your overall wellbeing for life-long change?

_____

_____

WEEK 9

You've nearly finished the *10-Week Challenge*. Hang in there!

This is a good time to start thinking about how you plan to continue after you finish the *10-Week Challenge*. Ask yourself whether you feel ready to resume any activities you haven't done for a while. It's OK to start slowly and perhaps seek further information from your PD Warrior Instructor or health professional before hand. Ideally, you will continue performing PD Warrior exercises at home and at your local PD Warrior site, if you have one, but either way you need to focus on how to maintain the gains you've scored over the past eight to nine weeks.

We have created a range of support resources to help you continue in your PD Warrior program long-term. If you have not already purchased, or considered these options, it might be worth considering them now:

- Online 10 Week Challenge – perfect for when you need additional support
- Online coaching for more one-on-one tailoring and support
- DVD – Use this when you are going away or need some guidance

All of these items can be purchased by visiting the website products page

At the end of the ninth week, record your feelings about exercise and your efforts.

I feel:

_____

_____

_____

I achieved:

_____

_____

_____

I am most proud of:

_____

_____

_____

The activity or exercise that I most want to get back to or have started doing is:

_____

_____

_____

To resume this activity/exercise I need to:

_____

_____

_____

WEEK 10

Congratulations! This is your final week of the PD Warrior *10-Week Challenge*. You should be feeling fabulous and in more control of your Parkinson's than ever before.

It's time to reopen your activity diary again. How much activity are you doing this week? Hopefully you have been inspired to increase your level of regular exercise by this stage. Record all of your exercise, and the level of effort you put into it over at least three days this week.

Compare Week 1 and Week 6 with this Week 10. Do you see an improvement? Are you excited? Inspired? How does this improvement match with your feelings of control and quality of life? It is likely that you can see a good correlation between your activity logs over the different weeks and your subjective feelings of control. If you have made good progress, you have just found a really good reason to keep exercising!

Week 10 is also a good opportunity to review your goals. Have a look at the short-term goals you wrote down before you started. How many of those have you achieved? What are you still working on and what is your plan from here? If you are struggling for answers, remember, you are never alone as a PD Warrior. Please talk to your PD Warrior Instructor for answers, support, and advice.

At the end of this week, stand up and congratulate yourself. You made it! You did it! You deserve a big reward for completing the *10-Week Challenge*. You've glimpsed what you are capable of and the progress that your efforts have yielded. Impressive! Well done!

At the end of this *10-Week Challenge*, record your feelings and activities.

I averaged _____ minutes of activity/steps each day this week.

In the past 10 weeks, I have achieved the following goals:

1. _____

2. _____

3. _____

The best moments in the past 10 weeks have been:

_____

_____

_____

I plan to keep the gains I have made by doing the following;

_____

_____

_____

_____

10

PD Warrior Core Exercises

'Most people never run far enough on their first wind to find out they've got a second.'

William James

The PD Warrior core exercises in this book are an abbreviated version of the PD Warrior circuit that we run in the gym. Your step-by-step PD Warrior home exercise program is set up here with a warm-up to start, the 10 PD Warrior core exercises, followed by stretches to finish. Your PD Warrior program should take you about 20-30 minutes to complete each day. You should aim to do your PD Warrior exercises twice on most days. If you add to that an additional 30 minutes of an activity that you enjoy, such as walking, swimming, or cycling, for example, you will achieve all or close to the 60 minutes of exercise that we recommend per day. For video demonstrations of the PD Warrior core exercises, please visit our website, http://www.pdwarrior.com/how-to-get-started.

It is important to think about the principles underlying PD Warrior as much as the exercises themselves. If you learn the key principles that we talked about earlier in Chapter 4 and focus on your exercises being specific to you, high effort, frequent, powerful, complex, salient, and fun, you are ready to start getting creative in adding those principles to your everyday life and activities.

The principles of PD Warrior set it apart from other exercise programs. To truly appreciate how important they are, you need to apply them consistently, through nearly every one of your movements.

The 10 PD Warrior Core Exercises are:

1. Sky Reach
2. Overhead Ball Throw
3. '007'
4. Scarf Snatch
5. Penguin Waddle
6. Banded Side-Step
7. Ta-dahs
8. Stop and Squat
9. Over the River
10. Box Step

The Warm-Up

Your warm-up is important because it not only gets your muscles primed for exercise and helps avoid injury but also gets your head in the right space. You should start to feel warm in your muscles during the exercise and your breath should be slightly laboured. The warm-up is not simply about going through the motions. Yes, you start slowly, but the idea is to progressively increase your effort level.

Think of it as loosening up. Have fun with it. If you have a song you enjoy, put it on and dance around the room. Go for a five-minute power walk around the block, climb a couple of flights of stairs, or climb on a home exercise bike. Whatever you do, it needs to be for a minimum of five minutes to get your blood pumping and your muscles ready.

1. Sky Reach

Here we focus on trunk rotation and big shoulder and arm movements to improve the range of movement in your upper back, trunk, shoulders, and hands. It also helps with powerful functional reaching.

Equipment

A sturdy chair, preferably without arm rests

Precautions

If you have any problems with your lower back, start slowly to avoid any injury. If you find it difficult to reach all the way to the floor and across your body, begin by extending your hand only as far as your opposite knee. You can also reach to an upturned tissue box or other target that is midway between your knee and the floor. Try and progress down your shin as you improve and as you feel more comfortable with the movement.

How to

Take a seat. During this exercise, visualise yourself as feeling powerful and strong. Now, spread your feet apart in a wide, supportive base. Holding on to the chair with one hand, reach across your body and down with the other hand and try to touch the floor on the outside of your foot. (If you can do this, well done!) Bring yourself back up into an upright sitting position. Now, using the same hand, reach upward across your body, towards the ceiling, fingers spread out as far as you can extend them. Look up at your outstretched hand. You should feel a powerful stretch across your chest, upper back, arm, and hand.

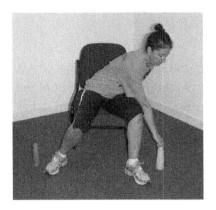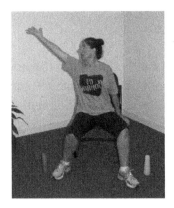

Cindy doing Level 1: Sky Reach – Start

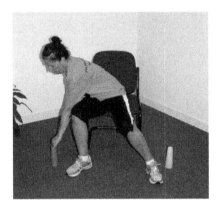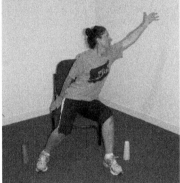

Cindy doing Level 2: Sky Reach – Finish

Repeat this exercise 9 times, reaching first to the floor, then sitting upright, and then reaching across to the ceiling. Now, switch hands and do another 10, reaching first to the floor, sitting upright, and then reaching towards the ceiling on the opposite side, all the time visualising yourself as powerful and strong. Can you detect any difference in how well you can reach on your left side versus your right?

Progressions

Level 1: Get used to the movement and start to add in some power.

Level 2: Move with as much power as you can. Each part of the movement should look and feel crisp and distinct from the other parts. Is your hand open wide, fingers splayed, at the top? Are you stretching up as far as you can? Are you extending beyond your base of support at the finish?

Level 3: Once you really get the hang of this exercise, begin introducing the mental tasking audio track that you downloaded from our *Get Started* page. Your primary focus should always remain on the motor task, and not the mental task.

2. Overhead Ball Throw

This exercise is designed to elicit force and power from the upper limbs and is especially good for people who experience slower, smaller movements and those who are tremor dominant. It works to improve your balance when throwing the ball and your control and coordination when catching the ball.

Equipment

A soft sponge ball, about 20 cm in diameter

Precautions

If you have a pre-existing shoulder injury, throw underarm instead, with your arms down in front of you. For those at a risk of back injury, make sure you do not arch your back excessively or place one foot forward of the other. This exercise can also be performed from a seated position.

How to

Face a solid wall, standing about two metres away. Place your feet about hip width apart to start. With the ball in your hands, bring your arms up over your head. Throw the ball overarm, using both arms together, and aim for a target above head height. Try to throw with enough force to catch the ball on the full, meaning hard enough that it returns to you. Remember your effort level should be at 80% so make sure you are standing far enough away from the wall to really make it challenging to catch the ball on the full.

Progressions

Level 1: If you are unable to generate enough force for the ball to return to you, try standing slightly closer to the wall.

Level 2: Once the exercise becomes easy, move further away from the wall and mix it up a little by standing in a tandem stance (as if standing on a tight-rope), single leg stand, or on a foam block.

Level 3: If you really get the hang of this exercise, introduce the mental tasking audio track, keeping your primary focus on the motor task, not the mental task.

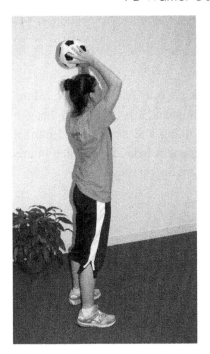 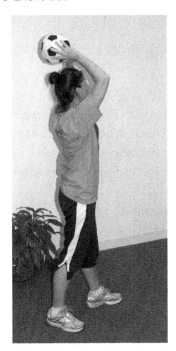

Cindy doing Level 1: Overhead Ball Throw

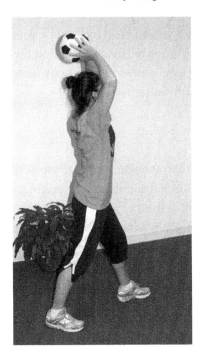 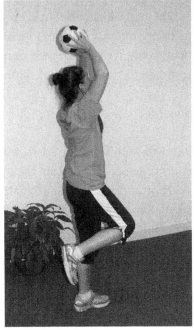

Cindy doing Level 2: Overhead Ball Throw

3. '007'

The focus of this exercise is to work on your trunk rotation. Many people with Parkinson's develop stiffness and loss of rotation through the trunk, which can affect your walking and posture and impact your balance as well. There is an element of balance indicated in this exercise, especially when you are changing direction.

Equipment

None (except a serious James Bond face)

Precautions

It is important to keep your hands together and to swivel on your opposite foot to protect your back. If you are prone to back pain, start with a smaller rotation, perhaps 45 degrees to each side instead of 90 degrees or more.

You may find it easier to keep your eyes and head focused on your hands as you turn in order to maintain your balance. If you find this too difficult, try keeping your gaze straight ahead as your body turns from side to side instead of shifting it from right to left.

How to

Start with your feet wide apart, wider than shoulder width. Clasp both hands together in a trigger grip, as if you are holding an imaginary handgun, and extend your arms straight in front of you, about shoulder height. Keep your eyes fixed on where you're aiming your gun. (Have some fun with this. We call this '007' because imagining yourself as a spy helps increase the intensity of the moves.)

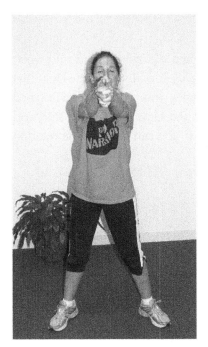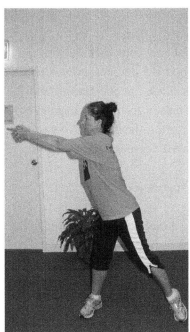

Cindy doing Level 1: '007'

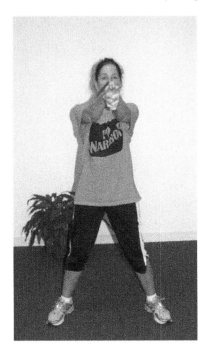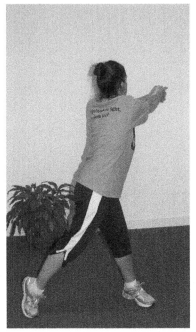

Cindy doing Level 2: '007'

Keeping your gaze on your aim, swing the gun around to your right, about 45 degrees, swivelling on your left foot if necessary. Hold that position for one second and then swing your 'gun' in outstretched hands in front of you again. Now, do the same on your left side, and return to facing front. As you improve, you can increase the rotation to 90 degrees and more.

Progressions

Level 1: Get the feeling of the movement, swivelling no more than 90 degrees left and right.

Level 2: Start putting more power into each turn, moving as far round as you can manage. Remember, your ideal effort level is working at 80%.

Level 3: When you really get the hang of this exercise, introduce the mental tasking audio track. Your main focus should always remain on the motor task, and not the mental one.

4. Scarf Snatch

This exercise focuses on arm swing and ballistic, powerful movements. This is a great exercise if your main symptom is bradykinesia (slow movement). You can increase the difficulty of the task easily as you progress.

Equipment

Two scarves, silk, tulle, or other lightweight fabric

Precautions

In the case of pre-existing shoulder injury, toss the scarves underarm and bend your arm at the elbow to gain force. In the case of poor balance, place a sturdy chair within easy reach.

How to

Holding a scarf in each hand, with your feet wide apart, throw one scarf directly up into the air, as high as you can. As the scarf floats down, snatch it back when it reaches shoulder height. The focus of this exercise is on the 'snatch', moving quickly enough to rip the scarf out of the air using an overhand motion. Do not wait for it to fall below shoulder height and do not try to catch it underarm. Now try doing it with the scarf in your other hand.

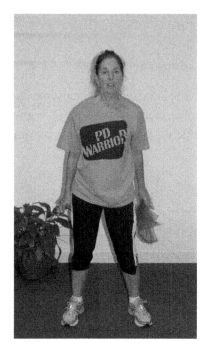
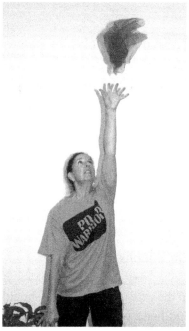

Cindy doing Level 1: Scarf Snatch

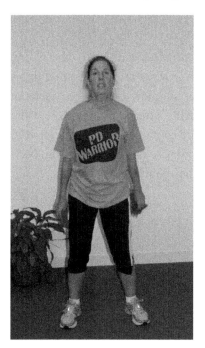
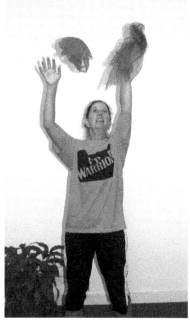

Cindy doing Level 2: Scarf Snatch

Progressions

Level 1: Repeat 9 times, using only the one hand and focusing on height of throw and speed of overhand catch. Then perform it with your other hand.

Level 2: Start to increase the speed of the snatch and the number of repetitions on each side. Try throwing both scarves, one in each hand, and seeing whether you can snatch the two scarves back with the same hand before they reach the floor. If this is not challenging enough, then you are not throwing the scarves high enough or snatching them fast enough.

Level 3: Once this becomes easy, introduce the mental tasking audio track, keeping your focus primarily on the motor task, and not the mental task.

5. Penguin Waddle

This exercise focuses on shifting weight and is a powerful way to improve your hip strength and dual tasking. It's a very helpful tool if you experience mild episodes of freezing when walking, not to mention it's a great butt workout!

Equipment

Four agility dots or markers on the floor, spread equidistant, about a foot apart in a square shape

Precautions

If you find yourself getting dizzy, try pausing after each square rotation. You might also want to place a sturdy chair at either side of the square to grab onto.

How to

Stand with your feet on the back two dots, arms at your sides, and practice shifting your weight from one dot (foot) fully to the other. As your weight shifts even more from one foot to the other, start lifting each foot off the ground in turn. Your body must stay straight. As you improve at this, you should feel the muscles on either side of your hips doing a bit of work.

Once you have got the hang of the weight shift, start doing the weight shift stepping around the square in a clockwise fashion, turning in a circle, facing outwards, keeping your feet on the dots and your arms at your sides. You should feel like a penguin, waddling as you face each direction. Once you have done one entire revolution around the square and returned to your starting position, reverse and do the same, moving in an anticlockwise direction. Each time you step, you should be stepping to a new dot and alternating between your left and right legs.

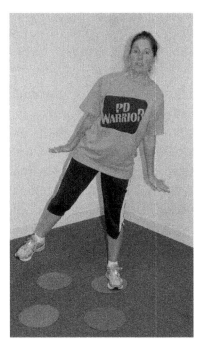
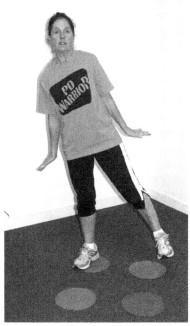

Cindy doing Level 1: Penguin Waddle

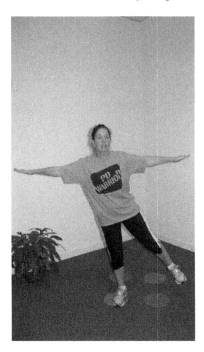
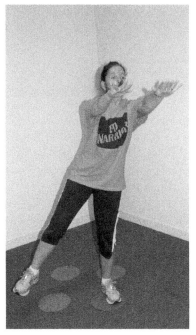

Cindy doing Level 2: Penguin Waddle

Progressions

Level 1: Perform penguin waddles in a clockwise and then anticlockwise direction with your arms at your sides.

Level 2: Do the penguin waddles just as you did in Level 1, and add the following arm combination. (Each step means a new arm movement.) When you take your first step, raise your arms up in front of you and extend them out straight so they are parallel to the ground; on the second step, pull them back down to your sides. When you take the third step, lift them straight out to the side, again parallel to the ground. When you take the fourth step, pull them back down to your sides. You might also want to move the dots outwards a bit to form a bigger box once you feel more comfortable with this.

Level 3: Once you really get the hang of this, introduce the mental tasking audio track, but maintain your primary focus on the motor task, not the mental task.

6. Banded Side–Step

This exercise focuses on posture, coordination, and upper limb resistance, and is terrific for getting the muscles in your back and arms to work hard.

Equipment

An elastic resistance band – start with low resistance and build up

Precautions

If you have a shoulder injury, keep your arms low and your hands well below your shoulders. You should feel the muscles in your shoulders and upper back working hard, but it should not be painful.

How to

Start with your legs about hip width apart in a power stance. Grab each end of your resistance band. Take a large step out to one side and, at the same time, fully extend your arms out to each side so that the resistance band stretches across your chest and the length of your arms. When you are fully extended, your chest should be out, your arms straight, and your hands slightly back behind your shoulders. Hold this position briefly and then release the tension of the band, pulling both arms into your chest as you draw your feet back to the starting position. If you have enough space, repeat this sidestepping across the length of the room. At the end, reverse direction and repeat the banded arms, leading with the other leg. If you do not have the space, just take a large step out to the opposite side, perform the stretch, and bring the leading leg back in to hip width apart, the starting position.

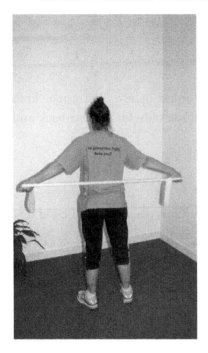
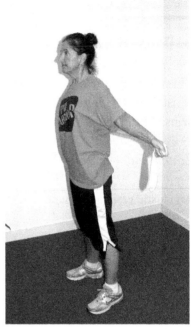

Cindy doing Level 1: Banded Side-Step

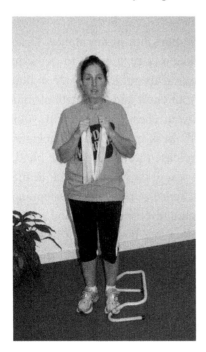
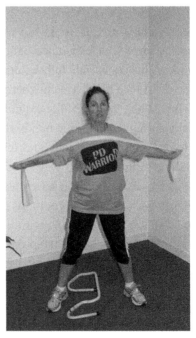

Cindy doing Level 2 : Banded Side-Step

Progressions

Level 1: Get the idea of the movement, focusing on achieving a full arm stretch with a big side-step with each repetition. To make this exercise easier, try starting by stretching the resistance band across your back instead of your chest. This has the added benefit of stretching you out through the chest and feels great!

Level 2: Use a higher-level resistance band and increase the power of your side-steps by stepping over a hurdle or foam block. Concentrate on moving your hands back behind your shoulders and extending your chest forward. Make sure that you keep the movements distinct and separate, not a sloppy recoil on the return movement.

Level 3: Once you get the hang of this exercise, introduce the mental tasking audio track. Note that your focus always remains primarily on the motor task, and not the mental task.

7. Ta-Dahs

This exercise focuses on shoulder extension, stepping, and exaggerated arm movement, with an added balance and coordination component.

Equipment

Two scarves (silk or other lightweight fabric) plus a foam block or adjustable height hurdle

Precautions

Modify exercise as appropriate, if there is pre-existing injury. If there are concerns about balance, place a sturdy chair close by and start with one side only, using the other hand for support.

How to

Start with your legs hip width apart and a scarf in each hand. Starting with the right leg, lift the knee high and take a small but powerful step forward. As you step forward, extend each arm out directly in front of you and then sweep them out to each side, like you are doing a stage show Ta-Dah! Make sure that you get a good stretch across the front of the chest and move your arms with sufficient power to make the scarves float horizontally. Step back, bringing both arms together fully extended in front of you. Repeat, alternating legs, 9 times. Ensure that both upper and lower limb movements are powerful going out and coming back, using crisp and distinct movements.

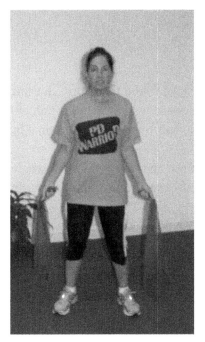 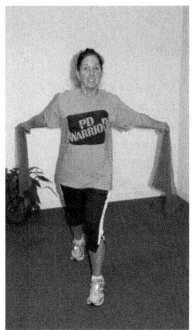

Cindy doing Level 1: Ta-Dahs

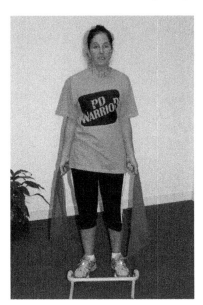 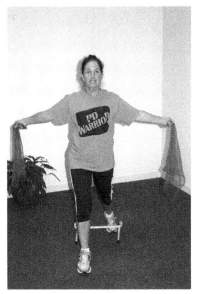

Cindy doing Level 2: Ta-Dahs

Progressions

Level 1: Get the idea of the movement and focus on achieving a full arm stretch and a high step forward with each repetition. To make this exercise easier, you can do this on one side at a time by holding onto a chair.

Level 2: Place a hurdle in front of you and step over it to increase the flexion at your hip and knee. Really exert yourself in a powerful way.

Level 3: When you get this exercise down pat, introduce the PD Warrior mental tasking audio track, always keeping your focus more on the motor task than the mental one.

8. Squat and Stop

This exercise focuses on power squatting to strengthen your legs and lower back and generate full extension and power in your arms and hands.

Equipment

A sturdy chair, preferably armless

Precautions

If you have difficulties with knee pain, start with slower squats, or half squats where you squat only halfway down. If balance is a concern, place another sturdy chair in front of you without obstructing your arms. In the case of pre-existing shoulder injury, change the arm position to a sideways movement and keep the hands lower than shoulder height at all times.

How to

Stand facing away from your chair, as if to sit down. Place your feet hip width apart and bend the knees slightly so that they project slightly ahead of your feet. Clench your fists and hold them against your chest, elbows tucked against your sides. Start to squat as if you intend to sit down, but stop just short of making contact with the chair seat. Do not sit down. The idea is that you will hover over the chair for a moment and then return to a standing position.

At the same time, perform a power movement with your hands. When you start to squat, bring your hands up into the 'STOP' position, open hands, fingers splayed, wrists extended, and arms reaching out in front of you, chest high, as if someone were running towards you and you wanted to stop them from barrelling into you. As you stand upright, your hands and arms pull back to your chest and your hands clench. Finish with your elbows tucked in.

Repeat 9 times and build up.

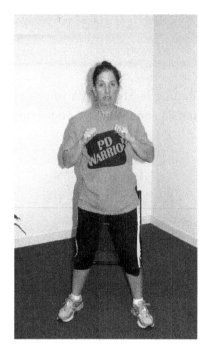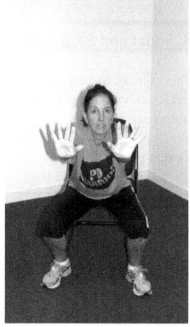

Cindy doing Level 1: Squat and Stop

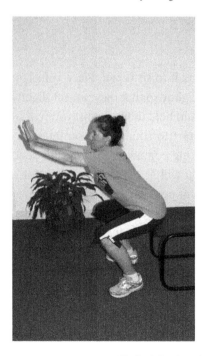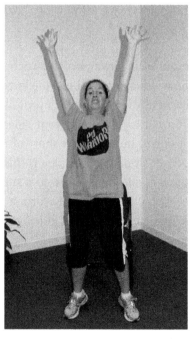

Cindy doing Level 2: Squat and Stop

Progressions

Level 1: Get comfortable with the coordination of the movement. Avoid tilting your upper body forward as you squat and make sure you stick your butt out as far back as you can to avoid overuse of your knees. Make sure you fully open your hands, stretch out your wrists, and move your arms with a powerful motion to indicate 'Stop'.

Level 2: To make this exercise more challenging, add a full shoulder stretch. Instead of just rising into a standing position, leap up from the squatting position, thrusting your splayed hands upward over your head, feet leaving the ground, and land in a standing position, arms fully stretching for the ceiling. Keep your knees slightly bent so that you land with soft knees, feet hip width apart, to reduce the load on your joints and better maintain your balance.

Level 3: Once you have Levels 1 and 2 of this exercise down pat, introduce the mental tasking audio track. Keep your focus mainly on the motor task, not the mental task.

9. Over the River

This exercise is excellent for coordinating big strides with powerful arm swings. It also helps with 180-degree turns.

Equipment

Small foam block or hurdle

Precautions

Do this exercise at your own pace. If the turns make you dizzy, slow down and take more time with each turn. If you have trouble with your knees or lower back, make your step smaller as you step over the hurdle.

How to

Place the foam block or hurdle on the floor in front of you. Lifting your knee high, step over the hurdle. If starting with your left leg, using an exaggerated standard walking arm motion, swinging your right arm forward with power and your left arm back as far behind you as you can. Keep your hands wide (fingers splayed) and open. Follow with the other foot so you have 'crossed the river'. When you are ready, turn around to face the hurdle again. Your 180-degree turn should be crisp and ideally achieved in no more than four to six steps. When you are ready, step back over the hurdle, this time leading with the other leg (right). Make sure to swing your arms with power and full range and bring your knees up high as you step over the hurdle.

Perform this 10 times in each direction and build up.

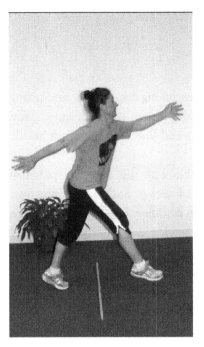 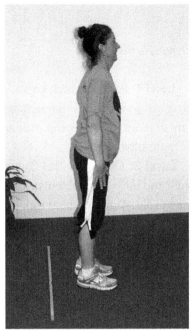

Cindy doing Level 1: Over the River

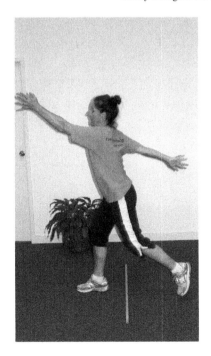 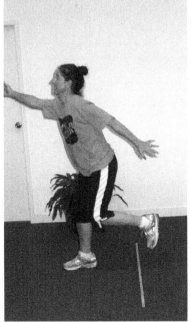

Cindy doing Level 2: Over the River

Progressions

Level 1: Focus on high knees, powerful big arm swings, and strong turns as you become familiar with the feel of this movement. You can start by just stepping over a marked line, rather than a hurdle or foam block.

Level 2: Once you feel comfortable with this exercise, can turn well, and have no problems with your knees or back, try leaping over the hurdle. Aim for height rather than distance. Use a powerful, large arm swing coordinated with the opposite leg, particularly exaggerating your back arm swing.

Level 3: Once you become proficient in this exercise, introduce the mental tasking audio track, always keeping your primary focus on the motor task over the mental task.

10. Box Step

This step focuses on your coordination, balance, and timing. It is a great exercise for challenging the coordination of your hands and arms as you combine it with a stepping exercise.

Equipment

Four agility dots or markers on the floor, spread equidistant, about a foot apart, in a square shape

Precautions

This exercise requires a lot of concentration. Make sure you feel steady on your feet before attempting this.

How to

Stand on the rear dots, one foot on each dot. Practice stepping forwards and backwards on the dots, starting with your right leg, in a box formation: forwards right, forwards left, backwards right, and then backwards left.

Once you achieve consistent timing and step accuracy and are ready to move to Level 2, add the arms as follows: as you step forward with your right leg, stretch your hands out in front of you, reaching forward and 'flicking' them open. As you step forward with your left leg, 'clench' them by making fists and drawing them to your chest. Now step backwards with your right leg and stretch your hands out again to reach forward and 'flick', and then step back with your left leg, closing your hands into fists again and bringing them to your chest in a 'clench'. With each step, you change your hand and arm position. Start slowly. You may find it helpful to practice the arm movements first before combining them with the steps.

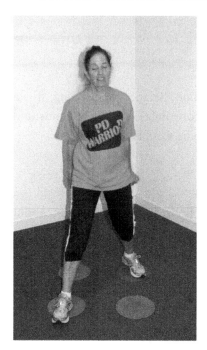
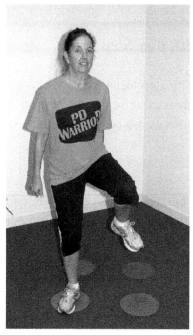

Cindy doing Level 1: Box Step

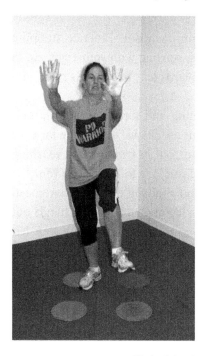
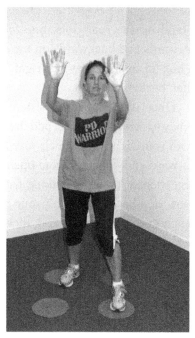

Cindy doing Level 2: Box Step

Progressions

Level 1: Focus on the legs first at this level. You want accurate timing and nice, high, firm steps: right, left, right, left.

Level 2: Add the arm movements described above. Alternate the flick and clench with each step. Make sure your hands are spread wide apart when you 'flick' and squeezed tight when you 'clench'. You may also want to widen your dots to make a bigger box to make it more challenging.

Level 3: Try stepping one complete box while leading with your right leg and then reverse direction, stepping one box leading with your left leg, all the while continuing the appropriate hand / arm movements. For a high-level box step, we often use agility stones to create a narrow base of support. For more information on agility stones, visit the website at http://www.pdwarrior.com/product.

Functional Tasks

Think about the activities you experienced the most difficulty with when you were filling in the self-assessment form. Write down your top 3 most challenging activities.

1. _____

2. _____

3. _____

Here are some techniques to consider for the tasks most people tend to have difficulty with.

Rolling in bed

If you have a lot of trouble rolling over in bed, think about how you do it. Are you putting enough effort into getting out of bed? Make your movements powerful and convincing and use a little momentum to get you up and over the side of the bed.

Unpacking the dishwasher

Here you simply may not be generating enough power in your movements. Short of smashing plates and glasses, you should be able to grab an item and move it swiftly up onto the kitchen bench. Start with larger items, like plates, and practice making an exercise out of each bend, grab, lift, and place on the bench. Each time you empty the dishwasher, you are potentially practicing 20 or more repetitions to generate more motor output.

Writing

Micrographia, or difficulty writing, is very common in people with Parkinson's. Your writing may be becoming smaller and more difficult to read. The good news is that, by performing most of the PD Warrior exercises, your writing should start getting easier and become more legible, even without actually practicing it specifically. If you feel you want to practice writing to improve it, grab a pen and some lined paper. Start by exaggerating the size of the characters so that they span double lines instead of single ones – make sure each letter crosses over two lines. As you get better at maintaining the size of your letters, try dropping down to a single line. Another handy tip to improve your writing if you see it getting smaller is to stop and practice 10 very hard and powerful hand flicks.

Cutting up food

If you have trouble cutting up your food, focus on making more powerful movements with your cutlery. The key is to think 'strong and powerful' with all your movements. You don't need to necessarily attack your food, but don't be shy or hesitant. Get stuck in!

Turning pages

This is one of my favourite activities to practice, probably because sometimes it ends in shreds of newspaper flying around the room. The next time you read a newspaper or magazine, be vigorous with each page turn. Up the ante and put more power into grabbing the page and flipping it over. Don't treat it with kid gloves, letting the page get the better of you by slipping through your fingers. If you tear the page the first few times, remind yourself that it's only newspaper. Make an exaggerated arc as you turn over the page. If you read a full broadsheet every morning, think of all the wonderful practice you're getting, generating more and more powerful movements every day!

Getting dressed

If getting dressed has become a challenge, if you have changed your clothing to avoid buttons and zips, it's time to revisit your wardrobe and drag some of those troublesome items out again. Choose an item you found particularly demanding. Is it a pair of tights you had trouble pulling up? A button-up shirt? Whatever the item, make it your mission to practice halving and quartering the time it takes you to get into it. Start by considering how much effort you put into your movements. Are they small and timid? Right then! Put in some elbow grease and make your movements more effortful, more deliberate. Even fine motor skills, such as doing up buttons, can be greatly improved by putting some more effort into your movements. Give it a try now. Imagine winning half your wardrobe back!

Opening doors

This is a test I like to get many of my clients to do. I casually ask them to walk into the next room, on the other side of a closed door. I am not interested in what's in the other room; I am interested in how they open the door without thinking about it. How do you open a door? Are you powerful and brisk? Do you stand with a nice wide base of support, or are you tentative and slow? Every time you open a door, think powerfully. View every door as an opportunity to drive greater effort and continue to improve your motor output.

Other tasks

Think of all the other tasks you once took for granted that you have either modified or had difficulty doing lately. There are any number of ways to improve how you handle activities that have become more challenging.

Stretches & Cool-Down

We have combined the stretches and cool-down together for practical reasons. Stretches themselves are unlikely to effect lasting changes to your posture, muscle length, or flexibility; however, they provide you access to a range of movement through which you can start actively moving. All of the PD Warrior core exercises have an element of flexibility and stretching built into them. If you combine those with the movements outlined in this stretching section, you may start feeling stronger and more powerful in your movements.

Table top

This is a powerful stretch for your shoulders, upper and lower back, and your hamstrings. Take your time moving into this stretch. If you find it too strong, start with a higher surface like a kitchen bench.

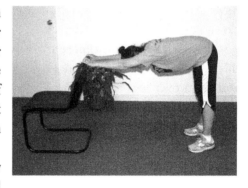

You will need a sturdy chair for this stretch. Stand behind the chair, place both hands on top of its back, and, holding on, walk backwards until you create a table top with your back. If you can, sink down into your shoulders, stretch through your upper back, and work to keep your lower back straight.

Hold this stretch for **20** seconds. When you are ready to come up, slowly walk forward towards the chair until you can push yourself back up into a fully upright position.

Power Trunk

This is a great stretch for your back and chest. It's what's known as a dynamic stretch, which means that you are not holding a position for any length of time, so take your time moving between the positions and try and stretch that little bit further each time. You will need a sturdy chair to do this exercise.

Start by facing the back of the chair. Place one hand on top of the chair back and take a big step back with the matching leg. Bend into the forward knee.

Gently extend your free hand as far behind you as you can in a stretch that opens you up through the chest and trunk and down into the hips. You may find yourself able to achieve an extension of more

than 180 degrees between your arms. As you progress, you can try turning your head to face the hand behind you. When you have stretched around fully, slowly come back to the starting position. I suggest you repeat this five times on one side before you swap over legs and hands and repeat on the other side.

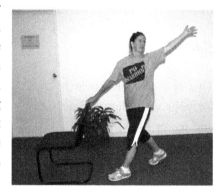

Superman

This is a great stretch for your chest and lower back. It encourages you to come up into a fully extended position.

Start by standing with your feet hip width apart. Place both hands behind you at your waist. Gently push your chest forward and extend up tall through your lower back. If you can maintain your balance, tuck your chin in and look up slowly towards the ceiling. Hold this position for 20 seconds and, when you are ready, slowly return to the starting position. You should feel taller for the stretch.

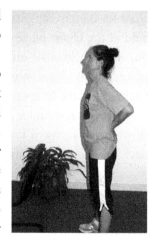

Log Roll

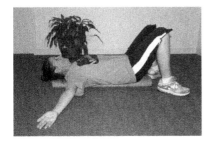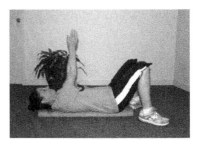

The log roll is a wonderful exercise to stretch out your upper back and chest. It is amazing how tall you can feel after this exercise. You need to take this stretch slowly as it can be quite intense the first few times. You also need to be able to get on and off the floor independently – if you have problems doing that, it's best to omit this stretch from your workout.

You will need a half foam roller for this exercise. Place the foam roller on the floor and sit on one end of the roller so that it extends behind you like a tail. Gently roll your spine down until you are lying on the roller and it runs along the length of your spine. Bend your knees to take the pressure off your lower back and keep your feet apart and flat on the floor to maintain balance.

If your head extends beyond the end of the foam roller, tuck a pillow beneath your head. Make sure to tuck your chin in so that you do not overextend your neck.

Raise your hands up to the ceiling and then slowly lower them out to each side, away from the body, like a cross. Your hands may not be able to touch the floor but you should feel a strong stretch across the front of your chest.

For your first time, I suggest holding this position for about a minute. As you get comfortable with this stretch, you can build up to 10 minutes each day.

To come out of the stretch, move your hands down to your sides. You can either roll sideways off the foam roller onto the floor or, if you are strong enough, roll yourself back up into a sitting position. Either way, gently raise yourself back up into a standing position.

11

Life after PD Warrior

Unite dedication with diligence because now the real work starts!

You have come so far!

Admittedly, it is hard to anticipate how well you will do in the PD Warrior program on your own. I know that, as a therapist in the PD Warrior hub, when I can motivate my clients in person through the *10-Week Challenge*, I can expect big things from them. My clients get results because we have a terrific support system, and there is no chance to slacken off. If you have not been to a PD Warrior site yet and done some of the sessions, I urge you to try. You may make great improvements without doing so, but it takes a lot more discipline and self-motivation to achieve the same results on your own. Either way, it's best to wait to read this chapter until after you have finished the PD Warrior *10-Week Challenge*.

So, now that you have completed the *10-Week Challenge*, how do you feel? You should be in top physical and mental condition if you have stuck with the program and should be seeing some encouraging gains.

Now is the perfect time to repeat your self-assessment measures, ideally within a week of finishing the *10-Week Challenge*. Do you remember the PDQ-8, Self-Assessment Parkinson's Disability Scale, six-minute walk test, and the Berg Balance Scale you looked at nearly three months ago? These are available in the back of this book, and if you registered for the *10-Week Challenge* on the website, you will have been sent some new assessment sheets. It's important that you don't sneak a peek at your previous pre-PD Warrior *10-Week Challenge* assessment scores before you do the re-assessment, as this can bias your results.

Once you have retaken the self-assessment and jotted down your scores, go ahead and pull out the original assessment you did. It's time to compare the scores.

Re-assessment test scores

How did you do? One of the assessment sheets should be a summary sheet. Insert your before and after results in order to see what you've accomplished after finishing the *10-Week Challenge*.

Let's start with the PDQ-8. Here we want to see that your score has dropped. The lower the score, the better in terms of measuring quality of life.

Now take a look at the SPDDS. We want this score to be lower this time around too. This measures your overall capacity to do tasks related to daily living.

In comparing the six-minute walk test, you should ideally be able to walk further than you did in the first round. How far can you walk now?

For the Berg Balance Score (BBS), the higher your score, the better your balance. Has your score risen since before starting the *10-Week Challenge*? The BBS can also be compared with other people your age to give you a benchmark.

Comparing the results

Even if your results stayed the same or you made more modest improvements in your outcome scores than you'd hoped, this is good news! Parkinson's is a progressive condition, so even managing to stay at the same level as you were three months earlier is a victory!

Everyone improves at different rates, with or without Parkinson's, and this can depend on many factors, including but not limited to how much time you spent doing your exercises and how frequently, how much effort you put in while doing them, and also how much support, motivation, and feedback you got during the program. It's no secret as to why personal training is a growing $500 million-plus industry. Most people do better when they are being watched, pushed, and encouraged - being held accountable on a daily basis. If you feel you worked hard but perhaps lacked sufficient feedback to help you to do your best, to achieve more than you could otherwise do alone, consider finding the PD Warrior site closest to you and booking in for a few sessions. Don't wait too long though, as you don't want to lose the ground you've worked so hard to gain.

If you're excited about how much you've improved, congratulations! That means you are feeling better, moving better, and thinking better. You worked hard and it's paid off. Go out and celebrate, and be sure to give yourself the reward you set.

Now what?

As I have said before, Parkinson's doesn't go on holidays - it's progressive and so must you be, always moving forward. You can't afford to rest now. You have to think long term, to focus on how to consolidate what you've learned over the past 10 weeks and apply your efforts to your daily routine. PD Warrior is designed to set you up for good long-term exercise behaviours and by now you should be working up to or have reached about *an hour of high-effort exercise a day*. Don't let all your achievements in increased fitness, strength, and hard work go to waste by letting things slide now.

You should be working up to or have reached about
an hour of high-effort exercise a day.

If you were looking forward to getting back to a sport, think about grabbing your buddy and trying it out. If you found a sport you enjoyed doing during the *10-Week Challenge*, by all means keep it going. Exercise is crucial for everyone in terms of keeping our bodies healthy and fit, and especially for those eager to fight the symptoms of Parkinson's. If it will help motivate you, think about continuing to record your sessions in your activity diary, especially the effort level you feel you are putting in. (It is always a good idea to re-calibrate your perceived effort level with feedback from your buddy.) Review your diary every couple of months to make sure that you are keeping your effort levels and activity levels up. Again, it's all about being pro-active! No-one else is going to do this for you.

Having finished the *10-Week Challenge*, keep doing the exercises that you found particularly helpful and make time for them in your daily routine. Visit the Facebook page regularly for updates and news about the program as well as keeping us posted on your results and gaining inspiration from the journeys of others. We are each other's biggest supporters!

Finishing the *10-Week Challenge* is a time of celebration but, if you're not careful, it can be too easy to let those few days off drag into one or two weeks, even a month. The longer the pause, the harder it will be to kick it back into high gear. You want to live every day, right? Then you owe it to yourself to work at it every day. Stay involved in the PD Warrior community and help others who are just starting out. It's amazing how the act of supporting others helps you to stay on track with your own program. If you are part of a broader Parkinson's support group, share your thoughts and experiences with PD Warrior with your group. Not only are you helping them, but surrounding yourself with like-minded people will also motivate you further. It's a win-win!

If your area lacks an accessible PD Warrior site and you have a community of people who are keen to do PD Warrior as a local circuit, let us know! The more people with Parkinson's who have access to a local site, the stronger the program will become. We need passionate and qualified PD Warrior Instructors, so if you have a good physio or exercise physiologist who might be interested in running the PD Warrior program in your area, please share with them how to get in touch with us. We run training programs regularly throughout the year for new instructors.

You are part of the PD Warrior Revolution, a revolution to change the way that Parkinson's is managed and treated now and into the future.

Parkinson's does not define you. PD Warrior can give you the control you've been missing and the hope you've lost. The choice is yours.

YOU ARE NOW A
PD WARRIOR FOR LIFE!

Record and Assessment Sheets

1. The 10–Week Challenge

Week 1

	Exercise	Repetitions							
1	Sky Reach								
2	Overhead Ball Throw								
3	'007'								
4	Scarf Snatch								
5	Penguin Waddle								
6	Banded Side–Step								
7	Ta–Dahs								
8	Stop and Squat								
9	Over the River								
10	Box Step								

Weekly Functional Training Tasks

	Task	Repetitions	Effort Percentage
1			
2			
3			

Week 2

	Exercise	Repetitions							
1	Sky Reach								
2	Overhead Ball Throw								
3	'007'								
4	Scarf Snatch								
5	Penguin Waddle								
6	Banded Side–Step								
7	Ta–Dahs								
8	Stop and Squat								
9	Over the River								
10	Box Step								

Weekly Functional Training Tasks

	Task	Repetitions	Effort Percentage
1			
2			
3			

Week 3

	Exercise	Repetitions							
1	Sky Reach								
2	Overhead Ball Throw								
3	'007'								
4	Scarf Snatch								
5	Penguin Waddle								
6	Banded Side–Step								
7	Ta–Dahs								
8	Stop and Squat								
9	Over the River								
10	Box Step								

Weekly Functional Training Tasks

	Task	Repetitions	Effort Percentage
1			
2			
3			

Week 4

	Exercise	Repetitions							
1	Sky Reach								
2	Overhead Ball Throw								
3	'007'								
4	Scarf Snatch								
5	Penguin Waddle								
6	Banded Side–Step								
7	Ta–Dahs								
8	Stop and Squat								
9	Over the River								
10	Box Step								

Weekly Functional Training Tasks

	Task	Repetitions	Effort Percentage
1			
2			
3			

Week 5

	Exercise	Repetitions						
1	Sky Reach							
2	Overhead Ball Throw							
3	'007'							
4	Scarf Snatch							
5	Penguin Waddle							
6	Banded Side–Step							
7	Ta–Dahs							
8	Stop and Squat							
9	Over the River							
10	Box Step							

Weekly Functional Training Tasks

	Task	Repetitions	Effort Percentage
1			
2			
3			

Week 6

	Exercise	Repetitions							
1	Sky Reach								
2	Overhead Ball Throw								
3	'007'								
4	Scarf Snatch								
5	Penguin Waddle								
6	Banded Side–Step								
7	Ta–Dahs								
8	Stop and Squat								
9	Over the River								
10	Box Step								

Weekly Functional Training Tasks

	Task	Repetitions	Effort Percentage
1			
2			
3			

Week 7

	Exercise	Repetitions							
1	Sky Reach								
2	Overhead Ball Throw								
3	'007'								
4	Scarf Snatch								
5	Penguin Waddle								
6	Banded Side–Step								
7	Ta–Dahs								
8	Stop and Squat								
9	Over the River								
10	Box Step								

Weekly Functional Training Tasks

	Task	Repetitions	Effort Percentage
1			
2			
3			

Week 8

	Exercise	Repetitions							
1	Sky Reach								
2	Overhead Ball Throw								
3	'007'								
4	Scarf Snatch								
5	Penguin Waddle								
6	Banded Side–Step								
7	Ta–Dahs								
8	Stop and Squat								
9	Over the River								
10	Box Step								

Weekly Functional Training Tasks

	Task	Repetitions	Effort Percentage
1			
2			
3			

Week 9

	Exercise	Repetitions							
1	Sky Reach								
2	Overhead Ball Throw								
3	'007'								
4	Scarf Snatch								
5	Penguin Waddle								
6	Banded Side–Step								
7	Ta–Dahs								
8	Stop and Squat								
9	Over the River								
10	Box Step								

Weekly Functional Training Tasks

	Task	Repetitions	Effort Percentage
1			
2			
3			

Week 10

	Exercise	Repetitions							
1	Sky Reach								
2	Overhead Ball Throw								
3	'007'								
4	Scarf Snatch								
5	Penguin Waddle								
6	Banded Side–Step								
7	Ta–Dahs								
8	Stop and Squat								
9	Over the River								
10	Box Step								

Weekly Functional Training Tasks

	Task	Repetitions	Effort Percentage
1			
2			
3			

Assessment Measures

	PRE Week 0		POST Week 10–12		FOLLOW–UP Week 26	
Date						
Ax Time						
	Secs	Steps	Secs	Steps	Secs	Steps
10mwt						
10mwt (MOTOR)						
10mwt (COGNITIVE)						
PDQ–8						
SPDDS						
BBS						
Activity log Mins / steps						
Challenge task						
	Metres	RPE	Metres	RPE	Metres	RPE
6mwt						
Observation gait / other						

Parkinson's Disease Quality of Life Questionnaire (PDQ–8)

Due to having Parkinson's disease,

how often <u>during the last month</u> have you ...   Please **tick one box** for each question

Task	Never	Occasionally	Sometimes	Often	Always or cannot do at all
1. Had difficulty getting around in public?	☐	☐	☐	☐	☐
2. Had difficulty dressing yourself?	☐	☐	☐	☐	☐
3. Felt depressed?	☐	☐	☐	☐	☐
4. Had problems with your close personal relationships?	☐	☐	☐	☐	☐
5. Had problems with your concentration, e.g. when reading or watching TV?	☐	☐	☐	☐	☐
6. Felt unable to communicate with people properly?	☐	☐	☐	☐	☐
7. Had painful muscle cramps or spasms?	☐	☐	☐	☐	☐
8. Felt embarrassed in public due to having Parkinson's disease?	☐	☐	☐	☐	☐

Please check that you have **ticked one box for each question**.

Thank you for completing the questionnaire.

Berg Balance Scale

Instruction: Can you do the following tasks?

For each item, score the lowest category that applies.

Sit unsupported with feet on floor		Can you sit to stand	
Able to sit safely and securely for 2 minutes	4	No hands, and stabilise independently	4
Able to sit 2 minutes under supervision	3	Stand independently using hands	3
Able to sit 30 seconds	2	Stand using hands after several tries	2
Able to sit 10 seconds	1	Minimal assistance to stand or stabilise	1
Unable to sit without support for 10 seconds	0	Moderate or maximal assistance to stand	0
Can you stand unsupported		Stand unsupported with feet together	
Able to stand safely for 2 minutes	4	Feet together independently, stand for more than 1 minute	4
Able to stand for 2 minutes with supervision	3	Feet together independently, stand for 1 minute + SB	3
Able to stand 30 seconds unsupported	2	Feet together independently, stand less than 30 seconds	2
Several tries to stand 30 seconds unsupported	1	Assistance to attain position, stand more than 15 seconds	1
Unable to stand 30 seconds unassisted	0	Assistance to attain position, stand less than 15 seconds	0
Stand unsupported with eyes closed		Reach forward with outstretched arm	
Able to stand 10 seconds safely	4	Can reach forward confidently more than 26cm	4
Able to stand 10 seconds with supervision	3	Can reach forward more than 13cm	3

Able to stand 3 seconds	2	Can reach forward more than 5cm	2
Eyes closed less than 3 seconds but stay steady	1	Reach forward but need supervision	1
Need help to keep from falling	0	Need help to keep from falling	0
Transfer from chair to chair		**Stand to sitting**	
Transfer safely with minor use of hands	4	Sit safely with minimal use of hands	4
Transfer safely with definite need of hands	3	Control descent by using hands	3
Transfer with verbal cueing and/or SB	2	Use back of legs against chair to control descent	2
Need one person to assist	1	Sit independently, uncontrolled descent	1
Need two people to assist or supervise to be safe	0	Need assistance to sit	0
Pick up object from the floor		**Look over left and right shoulder**	
Able to pick up object safely and easily	4	Look behind from both sides + weight shift	4
Able to pick up object but needs SB	3	Looks behind one side only – weight shift	3
Unable to pick up but keep balance	2	Turn sideways only but maintain balance	2
Unable to pick up and need SB	1	Need SB when turning	1
Unable to try and need max assist	0	Need assistance while turning	0
Turn 360 degrees, left and right side		**Alternate stepping on 26cm stool**	
Able to turn 360 degrees in less than 4 seconds	4	Safely complete 8 steps, in less than 20 seconds	4
Able to turn 360 degrees one side only, in less than 4 seconds	3	Safely complete 8 steps, in more than 20 seconds	3
Able to turn 360 degrees safely and slowly	2	Complete 4 steps without aid, + SB	2

Need close SB or verbal cueing	1	Complete 2 steps, needs minimal assistance	1
Need assistance while turning	0	Need assistance to keep from falling	0
Stand unsupported with foot in front		Stand on one leg (weakest)	
Tandem step independently, more than 30 seconds	4	Able to lift leg independently, hold more than 10 seconds	4
Foot in front, more than 30 seconds	3	Able to lift leg independently, hold more than 5 seconds	3
Small step in front, more than 30 seconds	2	Able to lift leg independently, hold more than 3 seconds	2
Need help to step, hold for more than 15 seconds	1	Attempt to lift leg independently, hold less than 3 seconds	1
Lose balance while stepping or standing	0	Unable to try	0

Total Score: _____

    49/56 = for those who walk without a stick indoors

    48/56 = for those who walk with a stick outdoors only

    45/56 = for those who use a stick indoors

    33/56 = for those who use a walker indoors

SELF-ASSESSMENT PD DISABILITY SCALE

Please rate the degree of difficulty you have doing each of these activities in general. If you use a mobility aid, please answer how well you would manage without the aid.

	1 Able to do alone	2 Alone but minimally difficult	3 Difficult or with help	4 Only able with a lot of help	5 Unable to do at all	Comment	N/A
1 Get out of bed							
2 Get up from an armchair							
3 Walk around the house							
4 Walk outside eg. to the local shops							
5 Travel by public transport							
6 Walk up the stairs							
7 Walk down stairs							
8 Wash face and hands							
9 Get into a bath							
10 Get out of a bath							
11 Get dressed							
12 Get undressed							
13 Brush your teeth							
14 Open tins							
15 Pour milk from a bottle or carton							

PD WARRIOR

		1 Able to do alone	2 Alone but minimally difficult	3 Difficult or with help	4 Only able with a lot of help	5 Unable to do at all	Comment	N/A
16	Make a cup of tea or coffee							
17	Hold a cup and saucer							
18	Wash and dry dishes							
19	Cut food with knife and fork							
20	Pick up an object from the floor							
21	Insert and remove an electric plug							
22	Dial a telephone							
23	Hold and read a newspaper							
24	Write a letter							
25	Turn over in bed							

Comments

SCORE:

Standard Tasks	Custom Tasks

Activity Log

Date	Activity	Mins	Reps	RPE*	Notes
TOTAL (count minutes / reps)					

* rate of perceived exertion

Goals

Short–term goals:

1._____ ☐ Achieved
2._____ ☐ Achieved
3._____ ☐ Achieved

Long–term goal:

4._____ ☐ Achieved

Reasons to Exercise:

1._____
2._____
3._____

I am doing PD Warrior because:

_____
_____
_____
_____
_____
_____
_____
_____
_____
_____
_____
_____
_____
_____
_____
_____
_____
_____
_____
_____
_____
_____
_____
_____

Performance Graph

(plot your progress here)

Challenge Task

_____

References

Ahlskog JE. Does vigorous exercise have a neuroprotective effect in Parkinson's disease? *Neurology* 2011; 77:288-294

Allen N, Canning C, Sherrington C, Fung V. Bradykinesia, muscle weakness and reduced muscle power in Parkinson's disease. *Mov Disord* 2009; 24(9): 1344-1351.

Allen N, Sherrington C, Paul S, Canning C. Balance and falls in Parkinson's disease: a meta-analysis of the effect of exercise and motor training. *Mov Disord* 2011; 26(9):1605-1615.

Archer T, Fredriksson A, Johansson B. Exercise alleviates Parkinsonism; Clinical and laboratory evidence. *Acta Neurol Scan*; 2011; 123; 73-84

Australian Institute of Health and Welfare 2012. Australia's health 2012. Australia's health series no.13. Cat. no. AUS 156. Canberra: AIHW.

Bello O, Sanchez JA, Fernandez del Olmo M. Treadmill walking in Parkinson's disease patients; adaptation and generalisation effect. *Mov Disord* 2008; 23 (9); 1243

Benedetti F Mayberg H, Wager T, Stohler C, Zubieta J. Neurobiological Mechanisms of the Placebo Effect. *The Journal of Neuroscience* 2005; 25(45):10390-10402

Beradelli A, Rothwell J, Thompson P, Hallett M. Pathophysiology of bradykinesia in Parkinson's disease. *Brain* 2001; 134: 2131-2146

Brauer S, Morris M. Can people with Parkinson's disease improve dual tasking when walking? Gait and Posture 2010; 31 : 229-233

Budden J & Sagarin B. Implementation Intentions, Occupational Stress, and the Exercise Intention–Behavior Relationship. *Journal of Occupational Health Psychology* 2007; 12 (4): 391–401

Cadet P, Zhu W, Mantione K, Rymer M, Dardik I, Reisman S, Hagberg S, Stefano G. Cyclic exercise induces anti-inflammatory signal molecules increases in the plasma of Parkinson's patients. *Inter J Molecular Med* 2003; 12: 485-492.

Campenhausena S, Bornscheina B, Wickb R, Bo¨tzelf K, Sampaiod C, Poewee W, Oertelb W, Siebertg U, Bergerc K, Dodela R. Prevalence and incidence of Parkinson's disease in Europe. *European Neuropsychopharmacology* 2005; 473 – 490

Canning C, Ada L, Woodhouse E. Multiple-task walking training in people with mild to moderate Parkinson's disease; a pilot study. *Clin Rehabil* e2008; 22: 226-233

Canning C, Allen NE, Dean CM, Goh L, Fung VSC. Home-Based Treadmill training for individuals with Parkinson's disease: a randomised controlled pilot trial. *Clin Rehabil* 2012; 26(9) 817-826.

Canning C, Sherrington C, Lord S, Fung V, Close J, Latt M, Howard K, Allen N, O'Rourke S, Murray S. Exercise therapy for prevention of falls in people with Parkinson's disease: A protocol for a randomised controlled trail and economic evaluation. *BMC Neurology* 2013; 28(S1).

Carne W, Cifu D, Marcino P et al. Efficacy of multidisciplinary treatment program on one-year outcomes of individuals with Parkinson's disease. *NeuroRehabilitation* 2005; 20: 161-167.

Carr J, Shepherd R. Neurological Rehabilitation: Optimizing motor performance. Oxford: Butterworth-Heinemann. 1987

Corcos D, Robichaud J, Leurgans D, Vaillancourt D, Poon C, Rafferty M, Kohrt W, Comella C. A two-year randomized controlled trial of progressive resistance exercise for Parkinson's disease. *Mov Disord* 2013; 28(9):1230-40.

Cramer et al. Harnessing neuroplasticity for clinical applications. Brain 2011; 134; 1591–1609

Cruise K, Bucks R, Loftus A, Newton R, Pegoraro R, Thomas M. Exercise and Parkinson's; benefits for cognition and quality of life. *Acta Neurol Scand* 2011; 123:13-19

Deloitte Access Economics. Living with Parkinson's Disease- update. 2011; http://www.parkinsons.org.au/ACT/AEReport_2011.pdf

Demirci M, Grill S, McShane D, Hallett M. A mismatch between kinaesthetic and visual perception in Parkinson's disease. *Ann Neurol* 1997; 41: 781-788.

Dibble L, Halc T, Marcus R, Droge J, Gerber J, LaStayo P. High-Intensity resistance training amplified muscle hypertrophy and functional gains in persons with Parkinson's disease. *Mov Disord* 2006 21(9): 1444-52

Duncan R, Leddy A, Cavanaugh J, Dibble L, Ellis T, Ford M, Foreman K, Earhart G. Comparative utility of the BESTest, mini-BESTest, and brief-BESTest for predicting falls in individuals with Parkinson disease: a cohort study. *Physical Therapy* 2013 Apr; Vol. 93 (4), pp. 542-50

EbersbachG, Ebersbach A, Edler D, Kaufhold O, Husch M, Kupsch A, Wissel J. Comparing exercise in Parkinson's disease- the Berlin BIG study. *Mov Disord* 2010

Ellis T, Boudreau J, DeAngelis T, Brown L, Cavanaugh J, Earhart G, Ford M, Foreman K, Dibble L. Barriers to Exercise in People With Parkinson Disease. *Physical Therapy* 2013: 10.2522/ptj.20120279

Erickson K, Raji C, Lopez O, et al. Physical activtity predicts gray matter volume in late adulthood: The Cardiovascular Health Study. *Neurology* 2010; 75:1415–1422.

Fabian D, Rafferty M, Robichaud J, Prodoehl J, Kohrt W, Vaillancourt D, Corcos D. Progressive Resistance Exercise and Parkinson's Disease: A Review of Potential Mechanisms. *Parkinson's Disease* 2012; doi:10.1155/2012/124527

Farley B, Koshland G. Training BIG to move faster; the application of the speed-amplitude relation as a rehabilitation strategy for people with Parkinson's disease. *Exp Brain Res* 2005; 167 (3): 462-467.

Farley B, Fox C, Ramig L, McFarland D. Intensive Amplitude-specific Therapeutic Approaches for Parkinson's disease. Toward a neuroplasticity-principaled Rehabilitation model. *Topics in Geriatric Rehabilitation* 2008; 24(2):99-114.

Fisher B Wu A, Salem G, Song J, Lin C, Yip J, Cen S, Gordon J, Jakowec M, Petzinger G. The effect of exercise training in improving motor performance and corticomotor excitability in people with early Parkinson's disease. *Arch Phys Med Rehabil* 2008; 89 (7): 1221-9.

Frazzitta G, Maestri R, Uccelini D, Bertotti G, Abelli P. Rehabilitation treatment of gait in patients with Parkinson's disease with freezing: a comparison between two physical therapy protocols using visual and auditory cues with or without treadmill training. *Mov Disord* 2009; 24 (8): 1139-1143.

Frazzitta G, Maestri R, Bertotti G, Riboldazzi G, Boveri N, Perini M, Uccelini D, Turla M, Comi C, Pezzoli G, Ghilardi M. Intensive Rehabilitation Treatment in Early Parkinson's disease: A Randomised Pilot Study with a 2-year follow up. *Neurorehabil Neural Repair* 2014: (epub ahead of print)

Frazzitta G, Maestri R, Ghilardi M, Riboldazzi G, Perini M, Bertolli G, Boveri N, Buttini S, Lombino F, Uccelini D, Turla M, Pezzoli G, Comi C. Intensive rehabilitation increases BDNF serum levels in parkinsonian patients: a randomised study. *Neurorehabil Neural Repair* 2014: 28(2):163-168.

Frazzitta G, Bertolli G, Riboldazzi G, Marinella T, Uccellini D, Boveri N, Guaglio G, Perini M, Comi C, Balbi P, Maestri R. Effectiveness of intensive inpatient rehabilitation treatment on disease progression in parkinsonian patients: a randomized controlled trial with 1-year follow-up. *Neurorehabil Neural Repair* 2012; 26(2):144-150.

Fuller R, Van Winkle E, Anderson K, Gruber-Baldini A, Hill T, Zampieri C, Weiner W, Shulman L. Dual Task performance in Parkinson's disease: a sensitive predictor of impairment and disability. *Parkinsonism Relat Disord* 2013: 19(3):325-328.

Gray W, Hildreth A, Bilclough J, Wood B, Baker K, Walker R. Physical assessment as a predictor or mortality in people with Parkinson's disease: A study over 7 years. *Mov Disord* 2009; 24(13):1934-40.

Gobbi L, Olivera-Ferreira M, Caetano M, Lirani-Silva E, Barbieri F, Stella F, Gobbi S. Exercise programs improve mobility and balance in people in people with Parkinson's disease. *Parkinsonism Rel Disord* 2009; 1553: S49-S52

Goodwin V, Richards S, Taylor R, Taylor A, Campbell J. The effectiveness of exercise interventions for people with Parkinson's disease: a systematic review and meta-analysis. *Mov Disord* 2008; 23 (5): 631-40.

Hackney M, Earhart G. The effects of a secondary task on forward and backward walking in Parkinson's disease. *Neurorehabil Neural Repair* 2009: http://www.ncbi.nlm.nih.gov/pmc/articles/PMC2888719/pdf/nihms158841.pdf

He Y, Zhang X, Yung W, Zhu J, Wang J. Role of BDNF in central motor structures and motor diseases. *Molecular Neurobiology* 2013 Dec; Vol. 48 (3), pp. 783-93

Hirsch M. Community-based rehabilitation for Parkinson's disease: From neurons to neighborhoods. *Parkinsonism Rel Disord* 2009; 1553: S114-S117

Hirsh M, Toole T, Maitland C, Rider R. The effects of balance training and high-intensity resistance training on persons with idiopathic Parkinson's disease. *Arch Phys Med Rehabil* 2003; 84 (8):1109-1117.

Hirsh M, Farley B. Exercise and Neuroplasticity in Persons living with Parkinson's disease. *Eur J Phys Rehabil Med* 2009; 45: 215-229.

Hiyamizu M, Morioka S, Shomoto K, Shimada T. Effects of dual task balance training on dual task performance ability in elderly people; a randomised control trial. *Clin Rehabil* 2011;26(1):58-67

Hyman C, Hofer M, Barde YA, Juhasz M, Yancopoulos GD, Squinto SP et al. BDNF is a neurotrophic factor for dopaminergic neurons of the substantia nigra. *Nature* 1991; 350:230-2

Janssen H1, Ada L, Bernhardt J, McElduff P, Pollack M, Nilsson M, Spratt NJ. An enriched environment increases activity in stroke patients undergoing rehabilitation in a mixed rehabilitation unit: a pilot non-randomized controlled trial. Disabil Rehabil. 2014; 36(3):255-62.

Kelly N, Ford M, Standaert D, Watts R, Bickel C, Moellering D, Tuggle S, Williams J, Lieb L, Windham S, Bamman M. Novel, high-intensity exercise prescription improves muscle mass, mitochondrial function, and physical capacity in individuals with Parkinson's disease. *J Appl Physiol* 2014: 116(5): 582-92

Keus S, BLoem B, Hendriks E, Bredero-Cohen A, Munneke M. Evidence-based analysis of physical therapy in Parkinson's disease with recommendations for practice and research. *Mov Disord* 2007; 22 (4): 451-460

King L, Priest K, Salarian A, Pierce D, Horak F. Comparing the Mini-BESTest with the Berg Balance Scale to Evaluate Balance Disorders in Parkinson's Disease. *Parkinson's Disease.* Volume 2012 (2012), Article ID 375419, http://dx.doi.org/10.1155/2012/375419

Lord S, Godfrey A, Galna B, Mhiripiri D, Burn D, Rochester L. Ambulatory activity in incident Parkinson's: more than meets the eye? *Journal Of Neurology* 2013: Vol. 260 (12), pp. 2964-72.

Mak MK, Hui-Chan CW. Cued task-specific training is better than exercise in improving sit-to-stand in patients with Parkinson's disease: a randomised controlled trial. *Mov Disord* 2008; 23: 501-509.

Merholz J, Friis R, Kugler J, Twork S, Storch A, Pohl M. Treadmill training for people with Parkinson's disease. *Cochrane Library* 2010.

Middleton A, Fritz S, Lusardi M. Walking Speed: The Functional Vital Sign. *Journal of Aging and Physical Activity,* 2015, 23, 314-322

Miyai I, Fujimoto Y, Yamamoto H, Ueda Y, Saito T, Nozaki S, Kang J. Long-term effect of body-weight supported treadmill training in Parkinson's disease: a randomised controlled trial. *Arch Phys Med Rehabil* 2002; 83: 1370-1373.

Morris M, Hylton B. Menz, PhD1 , Jennifer L. McGinley, PhD2 , Jennifer J. Watts, MComm (Ec)3 , Frances E. Huxham, PhD1 , Anna T. Murphy, PhD4 , Mary E. Danoudis, MPT1 , and Robert Iansek, PhD1,4Morris M, Iansek R, Kirkwood B. A randomised controlled trial of movement strategies compared with exercise for people with Parkinson's disease. *Mov Disord* 2009; 24 (1): 664-71

Morberg b, Jensen J, Bode M, Wermuth L. The impact of high intensity physical training on motor and non-motor symptoms in patients with Parkinson's disease (PIP): A preliminary study. *NeuroRehabilitation* 2014: (Epub ahead of print)

Muller T, Muhlack S. Effect of exercise on reactivity and motor behaviour in patients with Parkinson's disease. *J Neurol Neurosurg Psychiatry* 2010; 81: 747-753.

Muslimovic D, Post B, Speelman J, Schmand B. Cognitive profile of patients with newly diagnosed Parkinson's disease. *Neurol* 2005; 65:1239-1245.

Natbony L, Zimmer A, Ivanco L, Studenski S, Jain S. Perceptions of a Videogame-Based Dance Exercise Program Among Individuals with Parkinson's Disease. *Games Health J* 2013: 2(4):235-239

Neuner-Jehle S, Schmid M, Grüninger U. The "Health Coaching" programme: a new patient-centred and visually supported approach for health behaviour change in primary care. *BMC Family Practice.* 2013, 14:100

Nieuwboer A, Kwakkel G, Rochester L, Jones D, van Wegen E, Williems AM, Chavret F et al. Cueing training in the home improves gait-related mobility in Parkinson's disease: the RESCUE trial. *J Neurol Neurosurg Psychiatry.* 2007; 78(2): 134-140

Nieuwboer A, Rochester L, Muncks L, Swinnen SP. Motor learning in Parkinson's disease; limitations and potential for rehabilitation. *Parkinsonism Rel Disord* 2009; 1553: S53-S58

Obeso J, Rodriguez-Oroz M, Benitez-Temino B, Blesa F, Guridi J, Roriguez M. Functional organisation of the basal ganglia: therapeutic implications for Parkinson's disease. *Mov Disord* 2008; 23 (Suppl 3):S548-S559.

Olanow C, Kieburtz K, Schapira A. Why have we failed to achieve neuroprotection in Parkinson's disease? *Annals Neurol* 2008; 64(Suppl):s101-S110.

Onla-or S, Winstein C. Determining the optimal challenge point for motor skill learning in adults with moderately severe Parkinson's disease. *Neurorehabil Neural Repair* 2008; 22: 385-395

Ouchi Y, Yshikawa E, Futatsubashi M, Okada H, Torizuka T, Sakamoto M. Effect of simple motor performance on regional dopamine release in the striatum in Parkinson's disease patients and healthy subjects; A positron emission tomography study. *J Cerebral Blood Flow Met* 2002; 22: 746-752.

Paul S, Canning C, Sherrington C, Lord S, Close J, Fung V. Three simple clinical tests to accurately predict falls in people with Parkinson's disease. 2013 May; Vol. 28 (5), pp. 655-62.

Popiolkiewicz V, McConaghy M, Scrivener K, Dean C. PD Warrior Program Evaluation: Participants' satisfaction, feedback and health status survey. [Unpublished]

Prochaska J, DiClemente C, Norcross J: In search of how people change: applications to addictive behaviors. *Am Psychol* 1992, 47:1102–1114.

Peterson A, Pederson B. The anti-inflammatory effect of exercise. *J Appl Physiol* 2005; 98:1154-1162.

Petzinger G, Fisher B, Van Leeuwen J, Vukovic M, Akopian G, Meshul C, Holschneider D, Nacca A, Walsh J, Jakowec M. Enhancing Neuroplasticity in the Basal Ganglia: The role of exercise in Parkinson's disease. *Mov Disord* 2010; 25(Suppl 1): S141-S145.

Pisani A, Centonze D, Bernardi G, Calabresi P. Striatal synaptic plasticity: implications for motor learning and Parkinson's disease. *Mov Disord* 2005; 20(4):395-402.

Pohl m, Rockstroh G, Ruckriem S, Mrass G, Mehrholz J. Immediate effects of speed-dependent treadmill training on gait parameters in early Parkinson's disease. *Arch Phys Med Rehabil* 2003; 84: 1760-1766.

Ridgel A, Vitek J, Alberts J. Forced, not voluntary, exercise improves motor function in Parkinson's disease patients. *Neurorehabil Neural Repair* 2009; 23(6):600-608.

Rochester L, Baker K, Hetherington V, Jones D, Willems A, Kwakkel G, Van WEgen E, Lim I, Nieuwboer A. Evidence for motor learning in Parkinson's disease: Acquisition, automaticity and retention of cued gait performance after training with external rhythmical cues. *Brain Res* 2010; 1319:103-111.

Rollnick S, Mason P, Butler C: *Health Behavior Change: a Guide for Practitioners.* New York: Churchill Livingstone; 1999.

Sasco A, Paffenbarger R, Gendre I, Wind A. The role of physical exercise in the occurrence of Parkinson's disease. *Arch Neurol* 1992; 49(4): 360-365

Soh S, McGinley J, Watts J, Iansek R, Murphy A, Menz H, Huxham F, Morris M. Determinants of health-related quality of life in people with Parkinson's disease: a path analysis. *Quality Of Life Research: An International Journal Of Quality Of Life Aspects Of Treatment, Care And Rehabilitation* 2013 Sep; Vol. 22 (7), pp. 1543-53.

Springer S, Giladi N, Peretz C et al. Dual-Tasking effects on gait variability: the role of aging, falls and executive function. *Mov Disord* 2006; 21:950-957

Steffen T.M. Age and Gender Related Test Performance in Community-Dwelling Elderly People: 6MW Test, BBS, TUG, and Gait Speed. *Physical Therapy* 2002; Vol.82, No.2, Feb

Studenski S, Perera S, Patel K, Rosano C, Faulkner K, Inzitari M, ... Guralni J. Gait speed and survival in older adults. *Journal of the American Medical Association* 2011; 305(1), 50–58

Tanaka K, de Quadros AG, Santo R, Stella F, Boggi L, Gobbi S. Benefits of physical exercise on executive functions in older people with Parkinson's disease. *Brain Cognition* 2009; 69:435-441.

Tomlinson C, Patel S, Meek C, Herd C, Clarke C, Stowe R, Shah L, Sackley C, Deane K, Wheatley K, Ives N. Physiotherapy intervention in Parkinson's disease: systematic review and meta-analysis. *BMJ* 2012;345:e5004 doi: 10.1136/bmj. e5004 (Published 6 August 2012)

van der Heijden G. Shoulder disorders: a state of the art review. In: Croft P, Brooks PM (eds). Bailliere's Clinical Rheumatology 1999; 13: 287–309.

Van Nimwegen M, Speelman A, Smulders K, Overeem S, Borm G, Backx F, Bloem B, Munneke M. Design and baseline characteristics of the ParkFit study, a randomized controlled trial evaluating the effectiveness of a multifaceted behavioral program to increase physical activity in Parkinson patients. *BMC Neurology* 2010, 10:70 doi:10.1186/1471-2377-10-70

Van Hedel H, Waldvogel D, Dietz V. Learning a high-precision locomotor task in patients with Parkinson's disease. *Mov Disord* 2006; 21(3): 406-411.

Wood B, Bilclough J, Bowron A, Walker R. Incidence and prediction of falls in Parkinson's disease: a prospective multidisciplinary study. *J Neurol Neurosurg Psychiatry.*2002;72(6):721-5.

Xu Q, Park Y, Huang X et al. Physical activities and future risk of Parkinson's disease. *Neurology* 2010; 75:341-348.

Yin H, Ostlund S, Balleine B. Reward-guided learning beyond dopamine in the nucleus accumbens: the integrative functions of cortico-basal ganglia networks. *Eur J Neurosci* 2008; 28:1437-1448.

Lightning Source UK Ltd.
Milton Keynes UK
UKOW05f0812050517
300569UK00013B/148/P